W9-AHI-974

The Economics of Health

AN INTRODUCTION

The Economics of Health
AN INTRODUCTION

John G. Cullis & Peter A. West

New York · New York University Press · 1979

Library of Congress Catalog Card Number: 79-50451
ISBN 0-8147-1377-7

Manufactured in Great Britain

Contents

Notes and references at the end of each chapter

Preface

This short text is geared to students of economics and social sciences in general, and of health care services in particular, who have successfully completed a first-year degree-level course in economics or its equivalent. The material discussed is intended to cover the major aspects of the economics of health care, although for reasons of limited space many important contributions are mentioned only briefly in the text. The material included reflects not only British health care concerns but also the wide spectrum of the literature written in English, although there is a bias towards the concerns of developed countries.

The book is divided into five parts. Part I, an Introduction, consists of three chapters and includes a consideration of the nature of health care as an economic good and a discussion of how the principles of economics can be used to make predictions about the appropriate role of the 'market' and the 'state' in health care provision. Part II concentrates on both the theoretical and the empirical aspects of the demand for health care. Part III presents in its two chapters an essentially theoretical approach to the supply of health care concentrating largely on economic models of hospitals and the estimation of hospital cost functions. Part IV is devoted to an indication of the importance, relevance and difficulties of applying cost–benefit and cost-effectiveness techniques in the field of health care. The final part comprises three chapters on public policy problems and health care systems and concentrates in the first two chapters on the problems of particular health care systems – Chapter 10 the British NHS, and Chapter 11 the US health care system. The final chapter presents a more wide-ranging discussion of the health care problems of developing countries.

It is to be remembered that the economics of health care,

as a subject in its own right, is a relatively new one, largely dating from the mid-sixties. Although the frontiers have been pushed out rapidly during this period there are still large areas of unclaimed and virgin wilderness which in part accounts for the sections of 'B road' material connecting stretches of 'A road' and some 'motorway' material in this text. It is hoped, nevertheless, that the text provides an accurate introduction to where the subject 'is at' now and a basis for an appreciation and full understanding of the products of extensive current research to come.

Acknowledgements

Although this is essentially a secondary source book, concerned not with new contributions to the literature on the economics of health care but rather with an exposition and ordering of the existing literature, we have attempted not to make it tertiary rate. If we have been successful in this then much of the credit goes to Ron Akehurst, David Collard and Tony Culyer, who read, commented on and attempted to make sense of the whole of the manuscript.

For comments on particular chapters and sections of this book we are grateful to Jim Butkiewicz, Mike Drummond, Steve Heasell, Julian LeGrand, Ray Robinson and Sam Weller. We are also grateful to Alan Williams and Jack Wiseman, who, with Tony Culyer, first introduced us to the economics of human resources while we were both research fellows on DHSS-financed projects at the Institute of Social and Economic Research in the University of York. Many insights have also been gleaned from regular attendance at the biannual meetings of the Social Science Research Council-sponsored Health Economists' Study Group (HESG). Arthur Walker's current bibliographies of health economics, circulated to HESG members, have been a valuable source of references. Despite all this help, we are sure errors of commission and omission remain which must unfortunately be considered 'all ours'.

Finally, we must thank Christine Robinson for her typing, and especially our wives for spiritual support throughout and practical help with typing and indexing.

to our families and those who have been both willing and able to buy this book at the market price

PART I
Introduction

1 Health, Doctors and Health Care Resources

> If our society wishes to be rid of the diseases, fatal and non-fatal, that plague us the most, there is really little prospect of doing so by mounting a still larger health care system at still greater cost for delivering essentially today's kind of technology on a larger scale. We will not do so by carrying out broader programs of surveillance and screening. The truth is that we do not yet know enough. But there is also another truth of great importance: we are learning fast.
>
> *L. Thomas* (1977, p. 46)

1.1 Introduction

The 1960s and 1970s have witnessed considerable expansion of the areas that are a recognised part of the domain of applied economics. The economics of human resources is one such novel area of study, and health economics in turn is one of its newest and most controversial branches.[1]

It has become traditional[2] for human resource economists, especially when discussing health care, to justify their intrusion into what the layman at least might consider a field in which they are ill-equipped to contribute anything sensible. We do not intend to break from this tradition, and so we attempt in this introductory chapter first to explain why there is no reason to exclude health care from the glare of economic analysis and second to indicate the growing importance of health care as a scarce resource-user. In the sections below mention is made of good and bad 'health'. No attempt is made to define rigorously what is meant by these terms, on the grounds that to date no really satisfactory definition has been agreed upon. However, health is something that people have an everyday understanding of, and this is sufficient for the purposes of this book. For the record, one of the most popular (and most widely criticised) one-line definitions is that provided by the World Health Organisation (1958) as 'a state of complete physical and mental and social wellbeing'. This is not to imply that the definition of health is an inconsequential matter because, as Williams (1977) has recently pointed out, the definition chosen has widespread consequences. For example, if health is defined simply in terms of being alive, then success will be measured by changes in life expectation and resources allocated to treatments that save and extend life rather than to those that simply alleviate pain, demonstrate concern for the ill, etc.

1.2 Health care and a hierarchy of wants

As pointed out by Fuchs (1972), one of the commonest arguments for excluding economics from health care matters revolves around viewing good health as an overriding objective that individuals have that takes priority over all other objectives. In economists' terms, the implicit view is that people have a lexicographic ordering of their wants and desires with their health as top priority; i.e., desires are ranked in priority and the second is pursued only when the first objective has been attained. Thus there is no possibility of a 'trade-off' between health and any other desirable goal. It only requires casual introspection to dispel this belief. It is clear that each day everyone (except the dangerously ill) makes choices that may influence adversely their expected health state. They implicitly trade off decreased health against increased benefits of other kinds. The smoker who smokes an additional cigarette is implicitly saying that the marginal benefit derived from that activity is greater than the marginal cost, which includes not only the price of the cigarette but also the discounted present value of the expected lost time (because of an earlier death) and general reduced fitness consequent on smoking an additional cigarette. The pedestrian who crosses the road at a busy junction rather than using an underpass is weighing the marginal benefit of the avoided time and trouble costs of using the underpass against the increased risk of injury or death by road accident.

A further example might be the use of seat belts. The marginal benefit of not using one comprises avoided time and trouble costs and the feeling that others might view you as a namby-pamby risk-averter. The marginal cost is an increased risk of death and injury should you be involved in a road accident. The fact that some people smoke (25 per cent of doctors in the UK – (DHSS, 1977)) or do not use underpasses or seat belts is ample demonstration that their overriding concern is not with their health or safety.

Few people, if any, seek to maximise their health and life expectancy *per se*. To do so involves sacrificing opportunities to eat, drink, play games, drive, etc. that at the margin may be a greater source of utility than an additional (expected) minute or hour of life. (For a discussion of how people 'choose' the length of their lives see Chapter 4.) Good health and a long life are two among many desirable goals in life, and for most they are not afforded a special dominance in any hierarchy of wants. It may be argued that people *ought* to maximise their health/longevity estimate, but this takes us away from the realm of positive economics, where the economist *qua* economist is amoral or incompetent as regards the question of how individuals should behave, and into the difficult area of normative issues. Note, however, that we are concerned if individuals who value the health of others are willing to pay to effect institutional changes or changes in other parameters that influence people's behaviour such that their preferences are brought into account (i.e. the internalisation of external costs or benefits – see Chapters 2 and 3). Economists who accept the Pareto value judgement that individuals are usually the best judges of their own welfare seek to analyse and bring about situations in which individual preferences backed by purchasing power dictate the pattern of output or production. They do not question the preferences thus revealed.

Having established that no special place is afforded health care by individuals over and above other goods or services available, it is necessary to consider other claims made on behalf of health care and its practitioners. These are that health care is an essential to life and must be allocated resources irrespective of any cost–benefit considerations, and that medical decision-makers act in the best interests of their patients and are uninfluenced by economic factors.

1.3 Medicine and health

The naïve view of health care is that it is essential, otherwise people will not recover from what ails them and may, if the illness is serious enough, die. Luckily for those people who do not or cannot visit doctors regularly, this is a wild misconception. The body has a remarkable capacity to cure itself. This principle is brought out vividly by the following passage from the 1971 Rock Carling Fellowship lecture where Cochrane, writing of his experience of patient care during his time as a prisoner of war in Germany, continues:

> [I]n the *Dulag* at Salonika where I spent six months. I was usually the senior medical officer and for a considerable time the only officer and the only doctor. (It was bad enough being a POW, but having me as your doctor was a bit too much.) There were about 20,000 POWs in the camp, of whom a quarter were British. The diet was about 600 calories a day and we all had diarrhoea. In addition we had severe epidemics of typhoid, diphtheria, infections, jaundice, and sand-fly fever, with more than 300 cases of 'pitting oedema above the knee'. To cope with this we had a ramshackle hospital, some aspirin, some antacid, and some skin antiseptic. The only real asset were some devoted orderlies, mainly from the Friends' Field Ambulance Unit. Under the best conditions one would have expected an appreciable mortality; there in the *Dulag* I expected hundreds to die of diphtheria alone in the absence of specific therapy. In point of fact there were only four deaths, of which three were due to gunshot wounds inflicted by the Germans. This excellent result had, of course, nothing to do with the therapy they received or my clinical skill. It demonstrated, on the other hand, very clearly the relative unimportance of therapy in comparison with the recuperative power of the human body. On one occasion, when I was the only doctor there, I asked the German *Stabsarzt* for more doctors to help me cope with these fantastic problems. He replied: 'Nein! Ärtze sind überflüssig.' ('No! Doctors are superfluous.') I was furious and even wrote a poem about it; later I wondered if he was wise or cruel; he was certainly right. [Cochrane, 1972, pp. 4–5]

Apart from therapy not being essential it is rather disturbing to find there are instances in which it either makes no difference or makes matters worse. In an article on randomised clinical trials[3] (RCTs) Ederer (1977) has summarised some of the results of RCT studies into positive and negative categories. A couple of examples of the latter relate to gastric 'freezing' and treatment for viral hepatitis. In gastric freezing, duodenal ulcers are treated using a costly machine to induce hypothermia. This treatment was introduced in the early 1960s but not evaluated until 1969, when in a randomised, double-masked (blind) trial of 160 patients the 'freezing' procedures were shown to be no better than a sham procedure with respect to secretory suppression, pain relief or number and severity of recurrences. In an evaluation of hepatitis treatment a double-masked trial was conducted where patients with viral hepatitis were randomly assigned to corticosteroid or placebo therapy. Although the treatment had been in use since the early 1950s, it was concluded that it did not increase the survival chances of patients and might decrease them.

Perhaps the most often quoted study in this context is that of Mather *et al.* (1971), who used an RCT to evaluate treatment for ischaemic heart disease. The study concluded that hospital treatment including a variable time in a coronary care unit was not superior to treatment at home. Indeed, it is possible that the knowledge of being in intensive care contributes to cardiac arrest by increasing stress. (Although this conjecture is untested).

The most savage attack on the role of doctors and therapies in ill health has come from Illich (1975, 1976). Fuchs (1974) christened the hospital 'The House of Hope', but if Illich and his followers are right the hospital (and health aid generally) ought to be dubbed 'The House of Dope'. Illich commences his critique *Limits to Medicine* . . . (1976) with the words 'The medical establishment has become a major threat to health.' The threat comes in the form of *iatrogenic* (doctor-generated) diseases. Such disorders take three forms: clinical, social and cultural. The first occurs when medical treatment itself produces ill effects, which may be more severe than the disease for which the treatment was prescribed. Many examples support this case: the number of children disabled in Massachusetts through the treatment of cardiac non-disease exceeds the number of children under effective treatment for real cardiac disease; one out of five patients admitted to a typical research hospital acquires an iatrogenic disease, sometimes trivial, usually requiring special treatment of some sort with one case in thirty resulting in death. In similar vein, Gould (1976), has reported that a medical specialist in the use and misuse of drugs suggests that even heart specialists use digoxin wrongly by committing their patients to a long-term course of therapy with the drug. The patients often develop symptoms of poisoning resulting in their coming under the care of a geriatrician – the heart specialist never sees the consequences of his inept handiwork.

Social iatrogenic harm represents a second-level impact of medicine that is detrimental to the quality of life. Here the concern is with the reduced emphasis on the health-giving aspects of the social and physical environment and increased dependence on the medical profession. This dependence is 'unhealthy' when it results in intrusions at important times of privacy such as birth and death and when check-ups lead people to be anxious about their health. Furthermore, it is argued that the development of sensational transplant techniques raises false hopes and that the certification of health states reduces the individual's responsibility for his own actions. For example, once a doctor's certificate has been acquired, an individual's absence from work or forced removal to an asylum become legitimised.

Illich's third and final form of iatrogenesis is the cultural form, which is 'the paralysing of healthy responses to suffering, impairment and death' (Illich, 1976, p. 42). His thesis is that the individual gains from coping with pain and adjusting to the possibility of early death. However, medicine with its attempts to reduce pain and intensively treat the old and dying robs people of the learning experience and even of a dignified end to their lives. Illich argues that these forms of iatrogenesis have become medically irreversible, with further medical intervention to correct for iatrogenesis simply generating further iatrogenesis. It is the negative self-reinforcing loop of bad effects that is *medical nemesis*. To be saved from medical nemesis medicine must be de-professionalised so that care of the ill is returned as far as possible to the community, away from the medical profession, and with medical budgets firmly in lay control.

Clearly, the Illichian critique of medicine opens up an enormous range of issues for debate, many of which are beyond the scope of this book. However, one particular area where his thesis of medical mismanagement of individuals' lives closely fits reality is that of diagnosis and prescription, issues to which we now turn.

For two sorts of reasons it may be difficult to identify a particular state of ill health. One relates to the widespread absence of unambiguous indicators of ill health and the other to difficulties in observing and interpreting test results. Cochrane (1972) has emphasised the difficulty of interpreting the results of tests (especially haematological and biochemical ones). Ideally, for diagnosis one would like two separate distributions for the value of any health status indicator, e.g. pulse, blood pressure, etc., of the sick and the 'healthy', as in Figure 1.1(a). Unfortunately, the outcome depicted

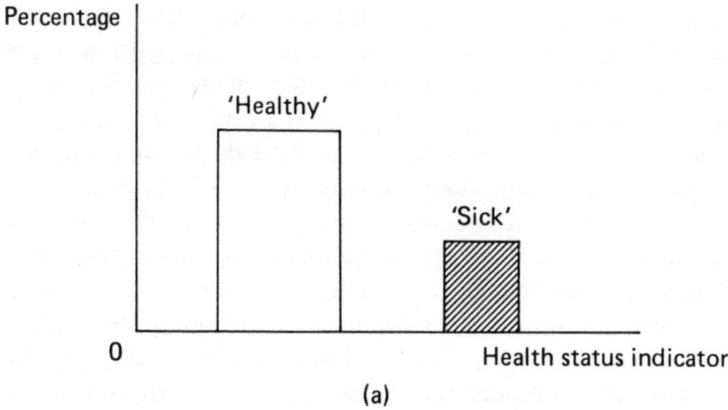

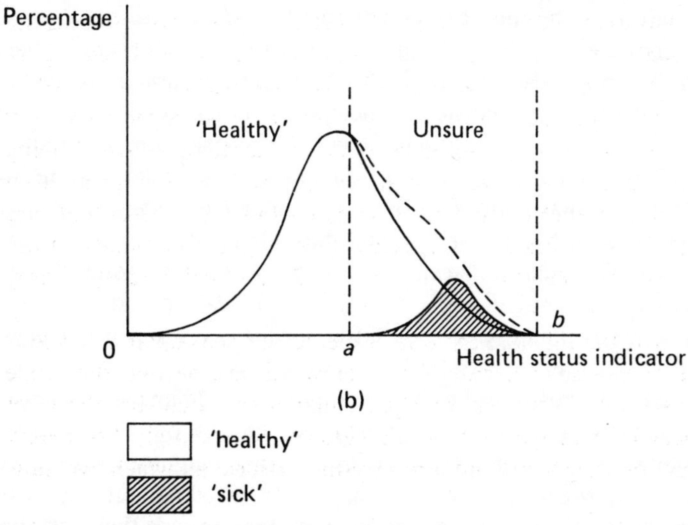

Figure 1.1 *Possible distributions of health status indicators in (a) naive 'theory'* and *(b) practice.* (*Source:* Cochrane, 1972)

in Figure 1.1(b) is common with an overlapping distribution of the characteristics of those who are 'healthy' and those who are 'sick', yielding a range *a* to *b* where it is uncertain (to a varying degree) whether the patient is indicated to be 'healthy' or 'sick' (i.e., skewed distributions of health status indicator and not bimodal ones are found in practice). The dilemma is well illustrated by essential hypertension. Drugs can be used to reduce blood pressure to normal. There is some (incomplete) evidence that prolonged treatment with anti-hypertensive drugs decreases the incidence of stroke as a consequence of hypertension. There is some less conclusive evidence that the incidence of coronary occlusion is also reduced. Thomas (1977) observed that on this basis there have been demands for large-scale screening so that the 10 million or more young potentially vulnerable people with hypertension in the USA will be treated on a life-long basis with complex drugs. However, many of the patients with essential hypertension would have the statistical probability of a normal life expectancy. For some, essential hypertension may in fact be 'normal'. The drawback is that those who will have cardiac, cerebral or renal complications associated with hypertension cannot be predicted. Therefore all hypertensives must be treated with drugs involving some known and probably some as yet unknown side-effects if the minority of patients is to be protected.

If it is difficult to get clear-cut indications of ill health, then diagnosis must also be a difficult and uncertain task. De Dombal *et al.* (1972) illustrated how difficult was the process of diagnosis even for common conditions. Their study compared computer-aided and human diagnosis in a series of 304 patients suffering from abdominal pain. The former's diagnostic accuracy of 91.8 per cent was significantly higher than that of the most senior member of the clinical team to see each case. The point is that, for acute abdominal pain, a common clinical condition with a relatively small number of possible disorders, even senior clinicians (in the General Infirmary at Leeds) were only 79.6 per cent correct in their diagnosis. Table 1.1 compares the diagnosis of senior clinicians with the final diagnoses. All entries off the principal diagonal (62 out of 304) represent wrong diagnoses. Shepherd (1972) has suggested however that the rate of correct diagnosis in the series was higher than appears on the grounds that non-specific abdominal pain was not a diagnosis.

Table 1.1 Diagnoses Made by Senior Clinicians in Charge of 304 Cases of Patients with Acute Abdominal Pain

Senior clinical diagnosis	1	2	3	4	5	6	7	8
Final diagnosis								
1 Appendicitis	75	1	—	6	—	—	—	3
2 Diverticular disease	—	2	—	1	—	—	—	1
3 Perforated duodenal ulcer	1	—	5	—	—	—	—	1
4 Non-specific pain	27	—	1	117	2	—	1	1
5 Cholecystitis	—	—	—	—	20	1	3	2
6 Small bowel obstruction	—	—	—	—	—	17	—	—
7 Pancreatitis	—	1	1	—	1	—	5	—
8 Other	3	1	—	1	—	1	—	2

Source: de Dombal *et al.* (1972)

It is also clear that the process of diagnosis varies widely between countries. Anderson (1976) and Jonsson and Newhauser (1975) studied one community general hospital in England, in Sweden and in the United States for comparative purposes. One of their findings related to the volume of various diagnostic tests per patient. The relevant data recorded in Table 1.2 make it clear that there is substantial variation that is unlikely to be removed even if the case mix were standardised, since evidence on diagnostic tests for acute myocardial infarction alone showed similar variation. Culyer (1976) added to the list of problems by pointing out first that diagnostic tests are not easily interpreted and then that, even when a diagnosis is arrived at, there is often no consensus on treatment. A surprising piece of evidence quoted by Culyer

Table 1.2 Numbers of Diagnostic Tests for All Patients by Patient-Days in Three Community Hospitals, by Country

	Country and year		
Test type	United States (1972)	Sweden (1972)	England (1973)
(1)	(2)	(3)	(4)
Laboratory tests/patient	7.0	2.7	5.0
X-ray examinations/patient	0.8	0.3	0.7
ECG's/patient	0.3	0.1	0.23

Sources: Anderson (1976) and Jonsson and Newhauser (1975)

to support the view that there are wide variations in treatment for identical conditions comes from the Sainsbury Committee's report on the pharmaceutical industry. For each of five common illnesses, 455 general practitioners prescribed over thirty different prescriptions, of which a small percentage (0.35 per cent) were toxic. Wade (1977) has also drawn attention to differences in the prescribing of drugs by doctors and remarked that

> The studies of the prescribing of hypnotic drugs and, more especially, of vitamin B12 preparations suggests that the prescribing of these drugs may be related not to medical needs of the community but to the traditions and habits of doctors or the expectations of people in the community. [Wade, 1977, p. 146]

Much of the variation in treatment may be harmless to the patient, but to the extent that treatments contribute to a cure it seems implausible that such a wide range of practice as that above would be cost-effective. However, the main point here is simply that treatment practices for given conditions do vary widely between doctors.

Fuchs (1974) has summarised the apparent consensus on the connection between health status and health care:

> True, advances in medical science, particularly the development of anti infectious drugs in the 1930's, 40's and 50's, did much to reduce morbidity and mortality. Today however, differences in health levels between the United States and other developed countries or among populations in the United States are not primarily related to differences in the quantity and quality of medical care. Rather they are attributable to genetic and environmental factors and personal behaviour. Furthermore, except for the very poor, health in developed countries no longer corresponds with *per capita* income. Indeed, higher income often seems to do as much harm as good to health, so that differences in diet, smoking, exercise, automobile driving and other manifestations of 'life-style' have emerged as the major determinants of health. [Fuchs, 1974, p. 6]

(For a theoretical discussion of the impact of income on the *demand* for health see Chapter 4.)

What then is the role of health care in developed countries? Dr R. E. Cook, quoted by Sifford (1977), has commented that health care is concerned with the five D's – *d*eath, *d*isease, *d*isability, *d*iscomfort and *d*issatisfaction. Of these five, health care does little at present to counter effectively the first and second except through public health measures. However, it has done a great deal to reduce disability, discomfort and dissatisfaction. Although it is true that the body has a capacity to cure itself of some diseases, that is not to say being (self-) cured without pain and discomfort is not a valuable service to non-Illichians.

There is a sixth 'D' that Cook might have added to his list. Health care is directed at *d*emonstration of concern, and this must be an important motive for some expensive procedures that are carried out with little impact on the health status of the patient. Intensive care units with continuous monitoring and laboratory tests are very expensive, yet a great proportion of people who receive such care do not survive twenty-four hours. Apart from any lives saved, the commodity provided in such circumstances seems to be demonstration of social concern, the knowledge that all that could have been done was done. Such a use of resources produces (*ex-post*) a commodity, 'peace of mind', in those related to the patient and for society at large. There is

Table 1.3 Measures of Health Status by Level of Per Capita GNP in Selected Countries[a]

Country (1)	*Per capita* GNP U.S. $ (2)	Infant mortality[b] (3)	Life expectancy[c] (4)
Upper Volta	70	180	39.0
Sudan	120	130	47.2
Bolivia	190	60	46.7
Ghana	250	156	43.5
Ecuador	310	87	59.6
Iraq	370	26	52.6
China (Republic of)	430	18	61.6
Cuba	510	28	72.3
Bulgaria	820	26	71.8
USSR	1400	23	70.4
Japan	2130	12	73.3
Israel	2190	24	70.5
USA	5160	19	71.3

[a] No specific year is given for the data in the source but they relate to the early 1970's.
[b] The number of deaths of children under one year of age per 1000 live births per year
[c] Expected length of life in years at birth

Source: World Bank (1975, Annex 2)

nothing inefficient about using scarce resources in this way as long as everyone is clear about what is being purchased and what is the foregone alternative, either in terms of other health care services or all other goods and services generally.

The emphasis above is on so called developed countries. But many developing countries have copied such patterns of health services in the face of very different health problems[4] (see Chapter 12). The illustrative statistics given in Table 1.3 are consistent with a development cycle hypothesis. At low levels of development, infant mortality is high and life expectancy is low, but they fall and rise respectively as income increases. At a GNP *per capita* of around \$500, life expectancy and the infant mortality rate level off, remaining almost constant as income rises. It is noticeable, for example, that the USA has a ten times greater GNP per head than Cuba and a slightly lower life expectancy.

1.4 Doctors and economic constraints

It has been pointed out that 'There seems to be an implicit tradition of assuming doctors (like civil servants?) are able, insightful, loyal, selfless, industrious servants of the public' (Culyer and Cullis, 1975, p. 18); that doctors are different from other men and women and are somehow untouched by the economic cost–benefit nexus that influences other people's actions. However, it is more realistic to assume that doctors are much like other people, and are not somehow paragons of virtue who operate independently of their economic environment.

This is not intended to be an attack on the integrity of those in the medical profession, but rather to argue that, like all other men, their actions are influenced by monetary and non-monetary rewards. This is perhaps the basic insight of recent literature on the economics of bureaucracy. A point often overlooked in introductory explanations of the theory of monopoly and competition is that both the monopolist and the perfect competitor have the same motivations – to maximise profit by producing where marginal cost equals marginal revenue ($MC = MR$). Although the monopolists appear as the black-hatted 'baddies' and the competitors as the white-hatted 'goodies', they are equally bad or good; it is just that the consequences of their similar motivations are economically harmful only in the former case. Hence it is no surprise to the economist that doctors' behaviour is influenced by the environment in which they find themselves. Economists expect doctors to maximise their own utility functions subject to the constraints they face. Elements in the utility function may be many and varied, but are likely to include income, work effort, peer group approval, public recognition, etc. Evidence makes it clear that it pays to devote considerable attention to the economic environment in which doctors and all other medical care decision-makers find themselves. For example, Lichtner and Pflanz (1971) examined the mortality rate for appendicitis and found it to be four times higher in the Federal Republic of Germany (FRG) than in any other country. The most probable reason for this is that the surgical procedure is performed in Germany three times more often than elsewhere. In attempting to explain why, the authors drew attention to the following environmental factors that influence the decision-making process of the specialist. First, having seen the patient only after a primary diagnosis by a family physician, the specialist faces a demand for an appendectomy that he may be reluctant to refuse unless he is certain that appendicitis is not the cause of the patient's problem; i.e., when in doubt take it out. Second, aside from possible fashions in surgery (which have occurred in the UK until relatively recently for tonsillectomy), the specialist may have a monetary incentive to operate, because of the requirement in the Federal Republic of Germany that applicants for surgical posts must have carried out a large number of appendectomies. Finally, hospitals may benefit directly from large numbers of appendectomy cases with a long period of recuperation (longer in the FRG than in comparable countries), during which the patient requires little care but pays a standard daily charge.

Although Lichtner and Pflanz have not claimed to be able to explain the high rates of appendectomy in the FRG, enough has been said to indicate the sort of factors that need to be considered. The process of excessive operations has been summarised in 'Bunker's Law', which states that if surgeons are in good supply, and if they are paid a fee per operation by patient insurance, there will not be any tonsils, appendices or Fallopian tubes left in the population (quoted in Anderson, 1976). Thus, although one might expect that the ethics of the medical profession would lead to a constancy of physician behaviour independent of the economic context, 'the literature on physician behaviour abounds with references to the responsiveness of physician practice behaviour to economic factors' (Evans, 1974, p. 165). Such responses form the basis both of Chapter 6 below, on supply, and Chapter 11, on current US health care institutions.

1.5 Resources devoted to health care

In this section an attempt is made to indicate the economic importance of the health care sector in developed and developing economies. Table 1.4 gives some limited data on the share of medical care expenses in Gross National Product (GNP). The general trend seems to be for health care to

(a) take an increasing proportion of GNP over time; and
(b) take a very different proportion of GNP in developing countries and developed countries.

There are several important reasons for expecting a rising proportion of health care expenditures in GNP; for example, the old and young consume relatively more health care services so that a changing population age structure might account for some growth.[5] Private insurance schemes and similar government schemes have made health care more accessible to many people. Technological change has been rapid in health care so that whereas ten or twenty years ago there was no therapy available for many conditions, today there is often a range of therapies, each expensive in terms of labour and capital inputs. These and other factors may well be relevant; however, Newhouse (1977) has recently had considerable success in explaining the quantity of resources devoted to health care in developed countries using only one explanatory variable – income *per capita*. In his study he addressed himself to the question of what determines the quantity of resources countries devote to health care. A simplified version of his approach follows.

For early 1970s data on thirteen developed countries Newhouse regressed *per capita* medical care expenditure upon GDP *per capita* yielding

$$M = -60.72 + 0.0788\,Y \qquad (1.1)$$
$$(2.57) \quad (11.47) \qquad R^2 = 0.92$$

Table 1.4 Health Expenditures as Percentage of GNP, Various Countries for Selected Years

	1950	1960	1960–1	1961	1961–2	1969	1970	1971	1972	1972–3	1973	1975
USA	4.6[a]	5.2[a]					7.1[a]					8.3[g]
UK	4.1[a]	3.9[a]					4.9[a]		5.06[b]			5.59[c]
Sweden		3.5[a]				6.4[a]						
Finland		3.5[a]					5.1[a]					
Italy		3.9[a]					5.2[a]	6.0[b]				
West Germany				4.5[a]		5.7[a]					5.26[b]	
Poland				3.7[d]							4.8[f]	
Czechoslovakia				3.6[d]							5.1[f]	
Tanganyika			2.5[d]				Tanzania			3.0[e]		
Kenya					3.5[d]							

Sources: [a] Maxwell (1974)
[b] Maynard (1975)
[c] *National Income and Expenditure, 1965–75*, London: HMSO
[d] Abel-Smith (1967)
[e] Gish (1975)
[f] Kaser (1976)
[g] Gibson and Smith Mueller (1976)

where M is medical care expenditure *per capita* and Y is GDP *per capita*. Over 90 per cent of the variance in *per capita* medical expenditure was explained by variation in GDP *per capita*.[6] (The figures in parentheses are t-statistics.) At the $3260.54 mean level of GDP *per capita* this implied an elasticity of care *per capita* with respect to GNP *per capita* of 1.31.[7] As a more rigorous test of the hypothesis that the medical care income elasticity is greater than unity (the conventional economic definition of a luxury good), Newhouse regressed the share of medical care expenditures on the reciprocal of GDP, i.e. effectively dividing the above relationship by GDP per head:

$$M/Y = \underset{(12.72)}{8.16} - \underset{(4.00)}{6883}Y^{-1} \qquad R^2 = 0.59. \tag{1.2}$$

Although the fit using the share of GDP as the dependent variable is inferior to the one using absolute values of the variables *per capita*, the coefficient of GDP was still significant.[8]

Two implications are drawn from the analysis, one of which is (fortunately) entirely in line with the discussion above. For developed countries at the *margin*, medical care appears to be a luxury good (i.e., income elasticity is greater than unity.) This is also indicated by time series data. If medical care is a luxury rather than a necessity, Newhouse suggested that the marginal unit of medical care does not produce an improvement in physiological health that will be reflected in mortality and morbidity rates. What then is being purchased? Following from the above discussion, it seems likely that a reduction in disability, discomfort and dissatisfaction is being secured.

In addition, rising income may permit additional tests, X-rays, etc., to confirm diagnoses rather than make them. Further, it seems clear that what high-income countries can afford is the feeling that all that is possible is being done for the ill irrespective of the expected change in health status. In Newhouse's words, 'countries that spend more may well buy more caring, but little additional curing' (Newhouse, 1977, p. 122).

The second implication is that, if income can explain a great proportion of the variance in *per capita* medical care expenditures, there is little role for other oft-mentioned factors. Hence the price paid by the patient, the method of doctor payment, etc., are not significant influences on the national expenditure on medical care. Newhouse explains this in terms of medical care being rationed, but not by the market mechanism; e.g., NHS expenditure is predetermined by Parliament. A corollary to this point is that richer countries can permit the health expenditures to rise and can have a more decentralised method of medical care. The latter may well be a good mechanism for delivering 'caring' type medical services. The picture in developing countries may or may not be as markedly different as one might expect. Cullis (1977) has constructed a sample frame of thirty-four developing countries for which data were available and carried out an analysis similar to Newhouse's. All the selected countries had a GNP (Y^1 below; Newhouse used GDP) of less than $1000 US. The source of the data was the World Bank (1975). The data differ from Newhouse's in that they relate to government health expenditure (M^1 below) rather than to private and governmental personal medical care expenditure but are similar in that they relate to the early seventies.

Regressing *per capita* government health expenditure on *per capita* GNP yields

$$M^1 = \underset{(1.23)}{-4.14} + \underset{(3.75)}{0.03Y^1} \qquad R^2 = 0.31. \tag{1.3}$$

Although this is an econometrically inferior result to equation (1.1), the income elasticity of demand based on this result at the mean of the data ($330.29) is 1.72, again indicating health care to be a luxury good.[9] Newhouse had avoided looking at data on developing countries for fear that differences in medical knowledge and type of disease would mask or distort any relationships present. Although it is clear that disease patterns are different in developing countries, it may well be that the broadly similar result can be attributed to medical technologies not being different over the world. That medical technology has an international currency has been observed with regret by Rifkin and Kaplinsky (1973), who have noted that many developing countries adopt medical care systems with capital-intensive delivery systems and a curative based type of care similar to developed countries. This is an issue taken up in Chapter 12.

1.6 Summary

The above has been a brief guide to some aspects of the relationships between resources devoted to health care and economics. In the early part of the chapter it was established that health care and health cannot be excepted from the attentions of economics on the grounds of their being an essential to life, or that decisions relating to health care matters are made in an hermetically sealed world free from the germs of cost and benefit considerations.

Some common misconceptions about the nature of health care and health were also explored. In the later parts of the chapter the growing relevance of health care economics is indicated by health care's importance as a percentage of GNP. Empirical evidence indicates health care to be a luxury good that at the *margin* may contribute little to physiological health, for developed countries at least. It was argued that national expenditure on health care was determined primarily by national income and not by concepts such as medical 'need'. This is not to imply that the price of health care, doctor payments systems, etc., are not important in determining *who* receives health care within a given total expenditure, but rather that medical science may be a major influence on costs but not necessarily on results.

In the chapters that follow we concentrate on the economic issues raised by this chapter. These concern the general nature of health and health care provision, a detailed examination of supply and demand, and a review of methods of evaluating health benefits. Finally, in the closing chapters we examine the issues and problems of health care provision in Britain and the United States and attempt to apply the lessons of health economics in a development context.

NOTES

1. We have in mind a common-sense interpretation of the term 'health care' meaning the services provided by doctors, nurses, hospitals, public health operatives, etc., whose object is to combat and prevent disease, restore and extend mental and physical fitness.

2. This is clearly one of those traditions that fall into the category initiated by the vice-chancellor of a new university, who felt his institution lacked 'traditions' so announced one morning that 'starting tomorrow morning it will be traditional to . . .'.
3. RCTs are concerned with applying the tools of statistical analysis to medicine in an attempt to separate objective evidence from clinical opinion by studying disease in defined groups rather than looking at individual cases. Bias is avoided by randomisation and 'masking' where the patient and/or the doctor is/are unaware of the treatment being administered.
4. The World Bank (1975) report that for developing countries the most widespread diseases are probably those transmitted by human faeces. The most common are intestinal parasitic and infectious diarrheal diseases, but also included are poliomyelitis, typhoid and cholera. Lack of community water supplies facilitates the spread of these diseases. The second major disease group affecting developing countries consists of airborne diseases, for example tuberculosis, pneumonia, diphtheria and bronchitis. The third major cause of mortality and morbidity in developing countries is malnutrition.
5. For example, Gibson, Mueller and Fisher (1977) have estimated that 44 per cent of US government expenditure for personal health care went to those under nineteen and those over sixty-five years of age. The former group accounts for 15 per cent and the latter 29 per cent. For a great deal of interesting statistics on and discussion of health care see Maxwell (1974).
6. The log-linear functional form yields only a slightly inferior R^2 but has the virtue of yielding income elasticities directly giving for the above:

$$\log M = \underset{(5.80)}{-7.37} + \underset{(9.86)}{1.56} \log Y \qquad R^2 = 0.90 \tag{1.1'}$$

$$\log M/Y = \underset{(2.15)}{-2.70} + \underset{(3.52)}{0.55} \log Y \qquad R^2 = 0.53. \tag{1.2'}$$

Equations (1.1), (1.2) (in the main body of the text) and (1.2′) are taken from Newhouse's article; however, (1.1′) was estimated by the authors from Newhouse's data. Equation (1.1′) indicates that a 1 per cent increase in *per capita* GDP results in a 1.56 per cent increase in *per capita* medical care expenditure. Equation (1.2′) indicates that a 1 per cent change in *per capita* GDP results in a 0.55 per cent increase in the share of medical care in GDP.
7. The formula for the elasticity in this instance is $dM/dY \cdot Y/M$ where $dM/dY = 0.0788$; mean level of GDP to the nearest dollar *per capita* is \$3260.54, which yields a value for M by substitution in equation (1.1) of 196.93 yielding a final elasticity of 1.3.
8. That a rising share of GNP implies a positive income elasticity of demand greater than unity is clear from the following. Assume $H = f(Y)$ where H is total expenditure on health care and Y is GNP. Our concern is with the share of GNP devoted to health care, (H/Y), and its rate of change as GNP rises.

$$\frac{d(H/Y)}{dY} = \frac{dH}{dY} \cdot \frac{1}{Y} - \frac{H}{Y^2}$$

$$= \frac{H}{Y^2} \cdot \left(\frac{dH}{dY} \cdot \frac{Y}{H} - 1 \right)$$

But $\frac{dH}{dY} \cdot \frac{Y}{H} = \eta_{YH}$ the income elasticity of demand for health care. Thus the growth of the share of health care expenditure with respect to GNP is only positive if $\eta_{YH} > 1$.

9. The log-linear functional form yielded the following result (t-statistics in parentheses):

$$\log M^1 = -4.97 + 1.10 \log Y^1 \qquad (1.3')$$
$$(4.22) \qquad (5.24) \qquad R_2 = 0.46$$

where 1.10 is the income elasticity of this constant elasticity functional form.

REFERENCES

ABEL-SMITH, B. (1967) *An International Study of Health Expenditure and its Relevance for Health Planning*. Geneva: World Health Organisation.

ANDERSON, O. W. (1976) 'All Health Care Systems Struggle against Rising Costs', *Hospitals*, Vol. 50, No. 19 (October), pp. 97–102.

COCHRANE, A. L. (1972) *Effectiveness and Efficiency: Random Reflections on Health Services*. (Rock Carling Fellowship Lecture) London: Nuffield Provincial Hospitals Trust.

COOPER, M. H. (1975) *Rationing Health Care*. London: Croom Helm.

CULLIS, J. G. (1977) 'Medical Care Expenditure: A Cross-National Survey: An Extension to Developing Countries'. University of Bath, mimeo.

CULYER, A. J. (1976) *Need and the National Health Service: Economics and Social Choice*. London: Martin Robertson.

CULYER, A. J. and CULLIS, J. G. (1975) 'Hospital Waiting Lists and the Supply and Demand of Inpatient Care', *Social and Economic Administration*, Vol. 9, No. 1 (Spring), pp. 13–25.

DE DOMBAL, F. T. *et al.* (1972) 'Computer-aided Diagnosis of Acute Abdominal Pain', *British Medical Journal*, Vol. 2, No. 5804, (1 April), pp. 9–13.

DEPARTMENT OF HEALTH AND SOCIAL SECURITY (DHSS) (1977) *Smoking and Professional People*, London: HMSO.

EDERER, F. (1977) 'The Randomised Clinical Trial', pp. 3–11 in Phillips, C. I. and Wolfe, J. N. (eds), *Clinical Practice and Economics*, Tunbridge Wells: Pitman Medical Publishing Co.

EVANS, R. G. (1974) 'Supplier-induced Demand: Some Empirical Evidence and Implications', pp. 162–73 in Perlman, M. (ed.) *The Economics of Health and Medical Care*. London and Basingstoke: Macmillan Press for International Economic Association.

FUCHS, V. R. (1972) 'Health Care and the United States Economic System', *Millbank Memorial Fund Quarterly*, Vol. 50, No. 2(1), pp. 211–37.

FUCHS, V. R. (1974) *Who Shall Live? Health, Economics and Social Choice*. New York: Basic Books.

GIBSON, R. M. and SMITH MUELLER, M. (1976) 'National Health Expenditures, Fiscal Year 1975', *Social Security Bulletin*, Vol. 40, No. 4 (February), pp. 3–20.

GIBSON, R. M., SMITH MUELLER, M. and FISHER, C. R. (1977) 'Age Differences in Health Care Spending, Fiscal Year 1976', *Social Security Bulletin*, Vol. 40, No. 8 (August), pp. 3–14.

GISH, O. (1975) *Planning the Health Sector – the Tanzanian Experience.* London: Croom Helm.

GOULD, D. (1976) 'How Doctors Generate Disease', pp. 105–09 in Carter, C. O. and Peel, J. (eds) *Equalities and Inequalities in Health.* London: Academic Press.

GOULD, D. (1977) 'The Springs of Suffering', *New Statesman*, Vol. 94, No. 2432, (28 October), pp. 574–7.

ILLICH, I. (1975) *Medical Nemisis: The Expropriation of Health, Ideas in Progress*, London: Marion Boyars.

ILLICH, I. (1976) *Limits to Medicine, Medical Nemisis: The Expropriation of Health*, London: Marion Boyars; also published 1977: Harmondsworth: Penguin.

JONSSON, E. and NEWHAUSER, D. (1975) 'Hospital Staffing Ratios in the United States and Sweden', *Inquiry* (Supplement) Vol. 12, No. 128 (June), pp. 128–37.

KASER, M. (1976) *Health Care in the Soviet Union and Eastern Europe.* London: Croom Helm.

LICHTNER, S. and PFLANZ, M. (1971) 'Appendectomy in the Federal Republic of Germany: Epidemiology and Medical Care Patterns', *Medical Care*, Vol. 9, No. 4 (July–August), pp. 311–30.

MATHER, H. G. *et al.* (1971) 'Acute Myocardial Infarction: Home and Hospital Treatment', *British Medical Journal*, Vol. 3, No. 5770 (7 August), pp. 334–8.

MAXWELL, R. (1974) *Health Care, The Growing Dilemma* (a McKinsey survey report). New York: McKinsey.

MAYNARD, A. (1975) *Health Care in the European Community.* London: Croom Helm.

NEWHOUSE, J. P. (1977) 'Medical Care Expenditure: A Cross-National Survey', *Journal of Human Resources*, Vol. 12, No. 1 (Winter), pp. 115–25.

PAGLIN, M. (1974) 'Public Health and Development of New Analytical Framework', *Economica*, Vol. 41, No. 4 (November), pp. 432–41.

RIFKIN, S. B. and KAPLINSKY, R. (1973) 'Health Strategy and Development Planning: Lessons from the People's Republic of China', *Journal of Development Studies*, Vol. 9, No. 2 (January), pp. 213–32.

SHEPHERD, J. A. (1972) 'Computer-aided Diagnosis of Acute Abdominal Pain', *British Medical Journal*, Vol. 2, No. 5809 (6 May), pp. 347–8.

SIFFORD, D. (1977) 'Medical Advice: Get Used to Pain', *Philadelphia Inquirer*, 28 August.

THOMAS, L. (1977) 'On the Science and Technology of Medicine', *Daedalus* (Proceedings of the American Academy of Arts and Sciences), Vol. 106, No. 1 (Winter), pp. 35–46.

WADE, O. L. (1977) 'Prescribing', pp. 141–60 in Phillips, C. I. and Wolfe, J. N. (eds), *Clinical Practice and Economics*, Tunbridge Wells: Pitman Medical Publishing Co.

WILLIAMS, A. (1977) 'Viewpoints on Health Research – An Economist's Viewpoint', *SSRC Newsletter*, 35 (October), pp. 9–11.

WORLD BANK (1975) *Health* (Sector Policy Paper). Washington DC: World Bank.

WORLD HEALTH ORGANISATION (1958) 'Constitution of the World Health Organisation Annex 1'. *The First Ten Years of the World Health Organisation*, Geneva: WHO.

2 Health Care as an Economic Good

> This section will list selectively some characteristics of medical care which distinguish it from the usual commodity of economic textbooks, . . . it is not claimed that the characteristics are individually unique to this market. But, taken together, they do establish a special place for medical care in economic analysis.
>
> *K. J. Arrow* (1963, p. 948)

2.1 Introduction

If those who have mastered a basic text in economics were asked what quantities of goods or services an individual would buy given his income or budget constraint, they would reply 'that bundle of goods and services that maximised the consumer's utility'. If pushed further, the apprentice economist would suggest that the consumption of each good would be extended to the point where the marginal valuation (*MV*) placed on the last unit of any good or service bought equals the price (*P*). To stop purchasing before this point would mean that the individual could increase his welfare by increasing the quantity purchased because the value of the additional unit to him is greater than the cost of acquiring it. Forgoing this gain is obviously irrational if maximum utility is the objective. To purchase beyond this point also implies irrationality, since the individual sacrificies more in the purchase of the additional unit than the value he puts on it; i.e., he makes himself worse off by buying it. So if we choose health care as a specific example of a service, we hypothesise that our 'economic man' would buy that number of units that equated marginal value (MV_h) with price (P_h). In Figure 2.1 this quantity is Oh^* units of health care per period. But if our budding

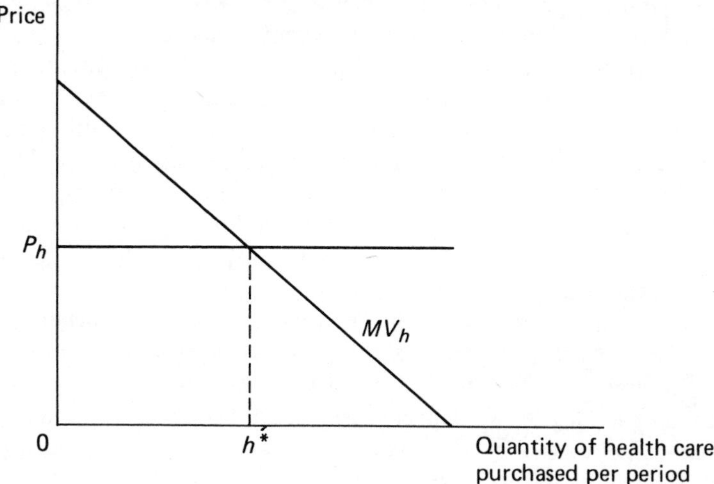

Figure 2.1 Utility-maximising purchase of health care

economist pursued his studies further he would spend much of his time discovering that in many cases this simple analysis is woefully inadequate. The health care market is one such case.

2.2 Classifying the benefits from improved health

Health care is one of a subset of goods and services, of which nutrition and education are also members, that provide both psychic and monetary benefits to consumers. The psychic benefits obviously derive from the curing of illness and the relief of pain which enhance the enjoyment of life now and in the future. The monetary benefits of health care arise because expenditures on health may possibly raise output and hence wages in future periods (as well as reducing future expenditures on health care). In short, health care can be seen as 'wealth producing as well as health producing' (Ministry of Health, 1956). To be more specific, improved health care generates four types of benefit for the individual who receives it.

(a) In the treatment period there is relief from the pain, suffering, anxiety, etc., consequent on ill health. (There may be a disbenefit if treatment makes the patient feel worse for the treatment time period, e.g. surgery.) This benefit is a non-durable consumption good providing utility in the current period only.

(b) In the periods following treatment there is a gain in the form of relief from the pain, suffering, anxiety, etc., that would have otherwise occurred without the provision of health care, i.e. the increased utility that comes from feeling healthy. This benefit is a durable consumption good lasting several periods. (b) differs from (a) in that it occurs in future periods, but is similar in that both provide increased utility 'pay-offs' to health care without any monetary benefits.

(c) In the periods following treatment there is the benefit in the form of a capital good, a capital good being one that yields utility indirectly as a part of a market production process. This capital good aspect is relatively easily quantified, being a monetary 'pay-off' measured by the increased production (and hence income) consequent on improved health status of the individual concerned.

(d) Recently Becker (1965) has emphasised that consumers are also producers combining own time with market-purchased inputs to produce fundamental commodities. A simple example might be combining purchased seeds, a garden plot and own (non-market work) time to produce 'home-grown' vegetables. Hence health care, if it increases the quality and quantity of time available for such non-market production, provides a capital good to be used in the non-market production process. (d) differs from (c) only to the extent that it is non-market gain and hence does not automatically have a monetary (pecuniary) value attached to it.

Expenditure on health care represents, to the extent outlined in (c) and (d), the construction of a capital good, and thus can be considered an investment in human capital with the market and non-market production type gains reaped in future periods being the return on the investment. In short, these are investment gains.

The categorisation of benefits to the individual from improved health into investment and consumption gains is somewhat arbitrary. For example, there is no reason why the non-durable consumption aspect (b) could not equally be termed an investment gain, with the return being in a non-monetary form, similar to the purchase of a work of art (see Section 4.3 below). For our purposes here it is sufficient that the reader knows what we have in mind by the terms used. With this aim in mind we have adopted (with minor adjustment to allow for Becker's pioneering work) Wiseman's (1963, p. 139n.) one-line definitions of the consumption and investment aspects of health care. The latter is 'the individual desire for good health because it brings a "pay-off" in output and income'. To allow for the 'pay-off' to be in non-market output and non-pecuniary income (c) will be described as pecuniary investment and (d) as non-pecuniary investment. Pecuniary investment will be discussed below because of the traditional emphasis placed on it. The non-pecuniary investment aspect will be included in the fuller discussion of the demand for health and health care in Chapter 4. The consumption aspect is 'the desire to live and be free from pain etc. for their own sake'. Hence (a) and (b) are termed consumption gains.

2.2.1 *Health as consumption*

Most economists are anxious to get away from the popular caricature of themselves as penny-pinching money-counters with no hearts and from the suspicion of the man in the street that economists concentrate largely on the monetary return to health and education (e.g., see literature on rate of return to education and early attempts at valuing life). But to an extent the man in the street is right. Most discussions of health pay lip-service to non-monetary aspects only because it is difficult to expand upon the obvious truth, 'good health is an end in itself' and equally difficult to quantify good health (see Chapter 8).

Recently Paglin (1974) has attempted to put non-monetary benefits on the same footing as monetary ones. His context is the developing country, where he argues that non-monetary aspects dominate monetary aspects because the effect of improved health on labour supply and marginal productivity is limited. Hence the whole of the emphasis of the analysis is concerned with making gains in life expectancy comparable to gains in real output. The consumer makes a choice between health care and other goods that may give a similar non-monetary return (e.g. foods that increase life expectancy) or satisfy desires. In Figure 2.2(a) the curves that spread out from the origin, i.e. AA^1, BB^1, CC^1 and DD^1, are production possibility curves showing the combinations of health care and other goods per capita that could be produced.

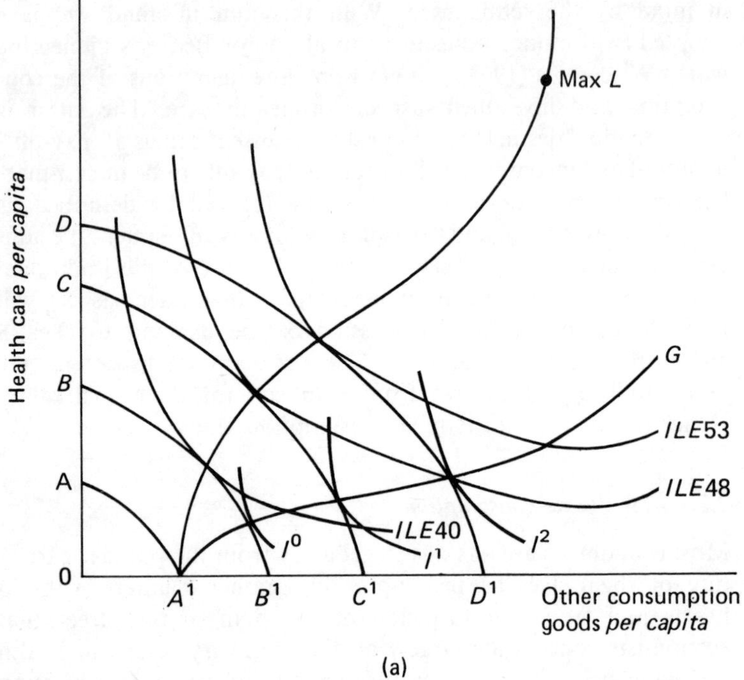

Figure 2.2 Health care and life expectancy

BB^1 represents a more developed economy than AA^1 and can, therefore, produce more of each. The convex curves labelled ILE40, ILE48 and ILE53 are iso-life expectancy lines indicating all combinations of *per capita* health services and other consumption goods that yield a given life expectancy e.g. forty years. The *ILE* contours flatten out and turn up, indicating that beyond some point additional consumption in the form of cigarettes, excess food and the other fruits of a sophisticated life-style have a detrimental effect on health. A given life expectancy can then be maintained only by purchasing more health care. A^1 Max L is the maximum life expectancy curve that links the points yielding the highest life expectancy for each production possibility curve (its tangent with an *ILE* curve). This becomes vertical at Max L, the point at which additional other consumption goods, even at higher levels of health care consumption, would have a zero or negative effect on life expectancy. OA^1 is the subsistence

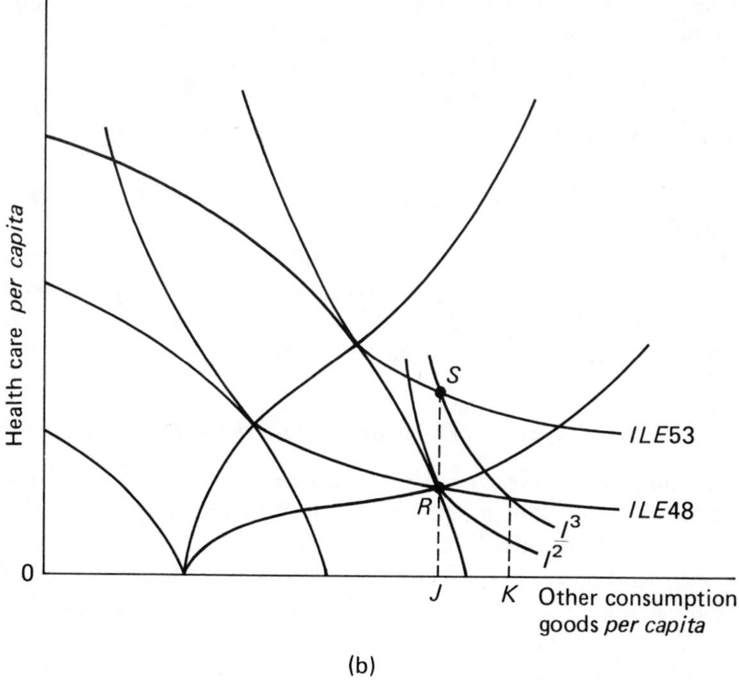

(b)

Figure 2.2 Health care and life expectancy

level of necessity intake where any further shift towards health care would increase mortality rates.

It is evident from casual introspection that individuals, or governments on their behalf, do not have as a maximand life expectancy alone.[1] If they did, A^1 Max L would be the equilibrium points. In fact, the curve A^1G is the equilibrium locus joining the points of tangency of community indifference curves I^0, I^1 and I^2 and the production possibility curves. Paglin used this framework to evaluate an improvement in life expectancy, say from forty-eight to fifty-three years, and make it comparable to an equivalent increase in material goods, as can be seen by looking at Figure 2.2(b), which is a simplified version of Figure 2.2(a). The indifference curves through R and S show the welfare gain (from I^2 to I^3) from an increase in life expectancy from forty-eight to fifty-three years at a consumption level of OJ other goods *per capita*. Its equivalent in material goods can be seen by finding the combination of the original life expectancy and additional goods, *OK*, that yields the same level of welfare as the improved life expectancy and the original level of other consumption goods *per capita*; i.e., *JK* in other consumption goods *per capita* is equivalent to an increase in life expectancy of six years. Although this analysis enables us to draw attention to the consumption benefits of health services, operationalising the model to measure these benefits is no easy task, and it is one that we defer until Chapter 8. In short, economists readily recognise that improved health increases utility quite apart from any pecuniary aspects. Economists do *not* argue that if the relief of pain and discomfort does not lead to increased market output it is irrelevant.

2.2.2 Health as pecuniary investment – the three 'D's'

As indicated above, the pecuniary aspect of good health is the desire for it because it increases the individual's output and earnings[2] (the classic work on this is Mushkin, 1962; also see Fuchs, 1966). If this occurs on any large scale it is possible to argue that devoting expenditure to health care creates sufficient resources to cover the expenditure itself and to generate a return. How can this come about?

The main possibilities are set out in Table 2.1. As can be seen from column (c), health improvements have a quantitative as well as a qualitative aspect, and it is the former that distinguishes health from the other major human resource investment, education.[3] Column (a), rows (1) and (2), indicate how the quantitative change in labour supply can be further sub-divided. Decreasing *death* rates effectively increases the size of the labour force, an absolute gain of man-hours. Decreasing the incidence of *disability* also increases the amount of labour time available by reducing the time lost from work because of ill health from a given labour force. The qualitative aspect, a reduction in *debility*, is easy to understand and represents a gain in working efficiency, but is much more difficult to measure than the quantitative aspects.

Lees (1960) tried to estimate the extent to which a developed economy could view health expenditures as a pecuniary investment by arguing along the following lines. Decreasing death rates, made possible by (alleged) improvements in food supply and public health, are likely to have been an important influence in the

Table 2.1 Potential Investment (Pecuniary) Benefits from an Improved Health Status of the Population

Description	Economic impact	Type of benefit
(a)	(b)	(c)
(1) A reduction in the number of premature deaths because of ill health	Absolute gain of man-hours	A quantitative aspect increasing the supply of man-hours.
(2) A reduction in the amount of disability or ill health to be found in the population	Relative gain of man-hours	
(3) A reduction in debility	Increase in productive capacity per man-hour	A qualitative aspect increasing output per man-hour.

eighteenth and nineteenth centuries for both demand and supply reasons. On the demand side an increasing population is likely to make for a buoyant market, hence stimulating the level of investment and perhaps making possible scale economies. On the supply side there would be the absolute increase in the work force outlined above. However, modern conditions are very different. Further substantial reductions in death rates are possible only among the old, who are likely to be increasing their consumption of health services as they fall foul of ailments requiring ever more sophisticated treatments. But since they are largely outside the labour force they are making no contribution to output as conventionally defined by the economist. Table 2.2 indicates life expectancies for selected countries showing that they already extend well beyond the normal working life for developed countries. Hence, further reductions in death rates generate no pecuniary return in developed economies.

A reduction in disability, and hence fewer working days lost, seems to be an alternative pecuniary return, but Lees has observed that, even if all work-days lost because of illness were eliminated, this would represent an increase in the total number of hours worked of only 0.5 per cent.

Table 2.2 Per Capita Gross National Product (GNP) and Life Expectancy in Selected Countries

Country	*Per capita* GNP[a] U.S.$	Life expectancy[b]
(A)	(B)	(C)
Burundi	60	39.0
India	110	49.2
Ghana	250	43.5
Republic of China	430	61.6
USSR	1400	70.4
Japan	2130	73.3
USA	5160	71.3

[a] World Bank, *World Bank Atlas* (1973) 'Population, Per Capita Product and Growth Rates', Washington: World Bank, pp. 6–14
[b] United Nations projections, 1973. Unpublished data: averages for 1970–75; defined as expected length of life in years, at birth

Source: World Bank (1975, Annex 2).

Finally, there is the third 'D', reduced debility. As suggested above, this possibility is difficult to measure, but given the widespread existence of social insurance to protect workers laid off through sickness, the presence of a worker at his place of work suggests that he thinks himself fit for work already (though clearly other social and economic pressures now influence his decision to attend work). Thus, it seems to be optimistic to expect a large 'pay-off' to be generated by reducing debility further.

Overall, we can conclude that pecuniary investment aspects do not provide a strong rationale for additional expenditure on medical care by the individual or the state. Ironically, there are reasons for supposing that this is also true for the so-called developing or Third World countries – but for very different reasons. Here there is likely to be considerable potential for decreasing premature deaths, disability and debility (see for example Table 2.2). However, as indicated in the previous section, this is of little relevance for developing economies because there is a surplus of available labour; hence Paglin's concern with the development of a non-pecuniary consumption framework for public health provision.[4]

Health care services, therefore, are a source of monetary and non-monetary returns and the rational individual in a market context would purchase that quantity of care for which the combined marginal value of these was equated with the marginal cost of health care. If all the usual theoretical conditions for a perfectly competitive market operated with respect to health care, we could perhaps end this book here. But this would be to ignore the manifold deviations of the reality of health care markets from such perfection. Therefore, we examine health care in detail in order to consider the reasons why health care is frequently not allocated in the same way as other services.

2.3 The characteristics of health care

There are many apparently diverse goods and services whose characteristics will prevent an efficient allocation in a competitive market. However, these characteristics typically fall into a relatively small set of categories. Traditionally these cover externalities, public goods, monopoly and merit wants. But for health care we might also add difficulties concerning choice under uncertainty.

2.3.1 Externalities

When a buyer and seller engage in a transaction it necessarily has implications for other people. Consumption patterns of potential buyers, who have been outbid, and production by other sellers will all change, though often in an infinitesimal way. However, these effects are not imposed on the other individuals. They arise because these individuals choose to act in a particular way. For example, a consumer who bids £4 for a good effectively states that he regards the good as equivalent, in terms of the utility he derives from it, to some other bundle of goods and services that he can buy for £4. If the market price is £4.50, which we assume he can afford, then he is not prevented from buying but chooses not to buy. Thus, the essence of market transactions is explicit choice. Externalities occur when a third party receives some benefit or suffers some loss without explicitly choosing to do so. An individual suffers from an adverse externality if smoke from a new factory damages his health and dirties his washing. Similarly, he benefits from an externality if his neighbour is inoculated against some disease as this will reduce his risk of contracting the disease.

The individuals making decisions that produce external effects will, unless forced by law or persuaded by money or other inducements, take no account of them. Thus, socially beneficial activities may be under-provided and socially harmful ones over-provided. Figure 2.3 illustrates this for the external benefits of vaccination

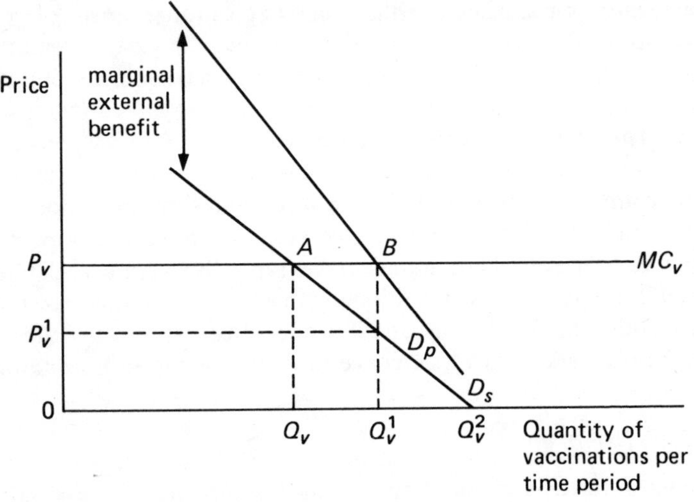

Figure 2.3 Polio vaccinations and external benefits

against a communicable disease, the most obvious, but, as will be noted below, not the most important, health externality. D_p is the (private) demand for inoculation based on the value of inoculation to the individual consumer. Vaccinations can be supplied at a constant price equal to marginal cost MC_v. The private market would reach equilibrium at point *A*. However, this is sub-optimal because individual private valuations of the benefits of vaccination ignore the benefits to others. The optimal outcome can be found by adding the value of these external benefits to the private valuation. This gives us a social valuation curve D_s where the *vertical* distance between D_p and D_s is the value of the marginal external benefit for each quantity of vaccinations. (In this example the two curves converge as the external benefit of an extra vaccination falls when the proportion of the population vaccinated rises.) The social optimum occurs at *B*, where the marginal social value of vaccinations equals the marginal cost.

This would only be chosen by individuals at the subsidised price of P_v^1.

The implication of the external benefits argument is that a private market system of provision, in which no mechanism exists to induce or coerce the transactors to take account of the external effects, will fail to achieve optimality, and that some form of public intervention is called for. Although the treatment of communicable disease is the form of health care for which such arguments are most often made, Lees (1960) has pointed out that the bulk of expenditures on health care today are not of this nature. By 1974 only 1 per cent of all cases treated in UK hospitals were concerned with infectious diseases. Of course, this may be the *result* of twenty-five years of market intervention in the form of a National Health Service, but it certainly reduces the force of the external benefit argument based on this physical external relationship.

Another form of externality argument has been developed by Weisbrod (1964), option demand. People have 'option' demands for facilities that they are not certain to use, for example hospitals; i.e., they would be willing to pay something for the knowledge that, should they put this book down, walk out into the street and get knocked down, there would be available capacity in hospitals for them to be treated. In a market in which the consumer pays only for the health care he receives, the owner of the hospital does not get any payment for the option benefit to the consumer. Thus, a hospital could close or reduce its size because of lack of revenue at a time when its existing size is providing considerable benefits that go unrewarded.

The adjustment in the market necessary to achieve the social optimum can take the form of public provision or of a system of charging for the option. The latter requires that the consumer buys the right to use the facility in the future. Such mechanisms are common in the finance of social and sporting organisations which provide a wide range of option benefits, but only to club members. Either public provision or pre-payment by the purchase of options can be used to secure the optimum, and so the argument does not imply market intervention. This will depend on other issues, such as the equity of different forms of finance.

Of greater significance for health care is the more subtle externality which recognises that people to some extent see themselves as members 'one of another' and are concerned with the amount of health care others receive. This externality may take several forms. Individuals may be concerned with those who in their view do not receive enough health care because of lack of income (the primary poverty argument), or because they are short-sighted or stupid and do not devote a sufficient share of their income (again in others' views) to health care. This is a secondary poverty argument. A third possibility is that people are concerned not with the absolute level of health care provision, but rather with the degree of equality with which it is divided among the members of society. The last pair of reasons has been the starting point for a number of major theoretical developments which form the core of the cases for intervention in the health care market. Therefore, they are discussed extensively in Chapter 3, which examines the intervention issue in depth.

2.3.2 Public goods

'Public goods' is the generic term of goods that yield a special set of external effects. The definition adopted here follows the definition set out, for example, in Musgrave and Musgrave (1976) and Peston (1972). This focuses on two characteristics that goods and services can possess, those of *rivalness* and *excludability*. The former simply means that one individual's consumption of a given good or service stands in a 'rival' relationship to another individual's; e.g., Stavros's consumption of a hamburger is rival to that of Kojak's because if Stavros eats a hamburger it reduces the remaining supply of hamburgers; the same hamburger cannot be eaten by Kojak. Excludability means, as its name suggests, that it is technically possible to exclude someone from the benefits of a good or service (note that for many public goods exclusion is possible technically but only at a cost so high as to more than offset the advantages). Thus, neither Kojak nor Stavros can consume a hamburger legally unless they (or a third party) pay for it. These two characteristics of rivalness and excludability enable the conventional market to work as an auctioning device, allocating goods and services to those individuals with the highest marginal valuations. Crudely speaking, it means that a hamburger is sold to the highest bidder. People will reveal their preferences for the hamburger and bid because they know first that it is rival, so that if it is sold to someone else then that hamburger will not be available to them, and second that it is excludable, so that if they do not pay the market price for a hamburger they will be physically excluded from consuming it. Most commodities have these characteristics of rivalness and excludability and are described as pure private goods which the market may allocate efficiently (though not necessarily equitably). However, if either or both of the characteristics illustrated above is absent it becomes difficult for the auctioning function of the market to operate. Figure 2.4 sets out the possible combinations of the two characteristics. In box 1 the characteristics of rivalness and excludability

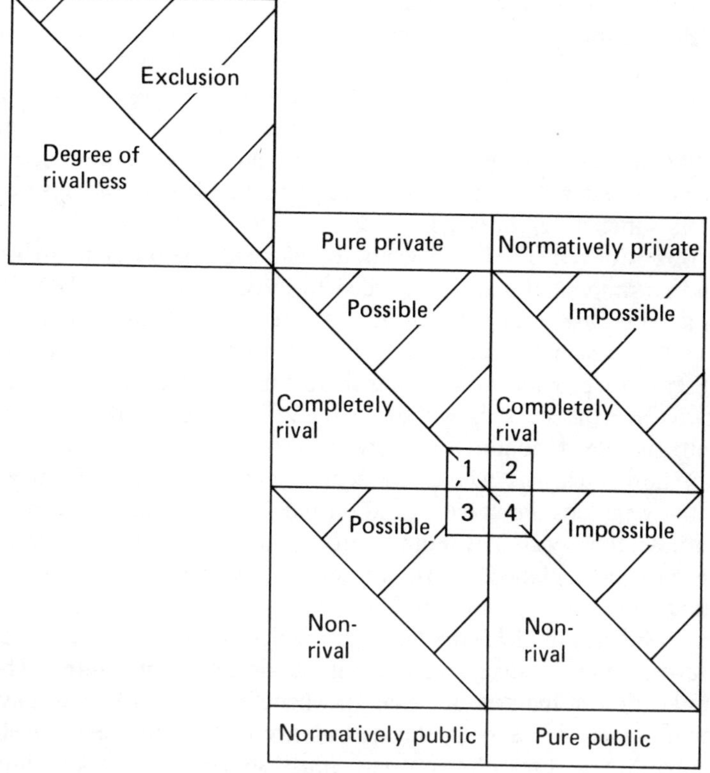

Figure 2.4 A classification of goods and services

apply and these commodities are pure private goods. What about boxes 2, 3 and 4? In all these cases the market runs into difficulties. In box 2 rivalness applies so that one individual's consumption prevents another individual's consumption but exclusion is not feasible. The importance of the latter is that it reduces the individual's incentive to bid for the good because it implies that he cannot be excluded from the benefits even if he does *not* pay. The usual example is the crowded city street; the space is rival, it cannot be occupied by two vehicles at the same time. It would be desirable to auction off the use of limited road space at times of overcrowding but because the technically efficient mechanism to exclude people is too costly the auction is not chosen (except in a Kantian world). In this case the good or service *ought* to be private and hence exclusion applied, but it is not realistic to try to do so – hence the description, 'normatively private goods'.

Box 3, the non-rival but excludable possibility, represents the 'normative public good'. Here it is possible to exclude people from the use of a facility, say an uncrowded bridge, at low cost by tolls; but because its use is non-rival as long as the bridge is uncrowded it would be inefficient to do so since some could be made better off by being allowed to use the bridge and existing users suffer no extra costs.

Box 4 covers pure public goods where the good is non-rival and no individual can be excluded from consuming. The benefits of a lighthouse or of national defence are the most cited examples. Lighthouses can be seen by all local shipping and the same quantity of service is provided to all. Thus there is an incentive to 'free-ride', to receive the benefits without paying for them, and a market will provide a quantity of service less than the optimum. As we showed earlier, where the social value of benefits from an activity exceeds the value placed on the activity by those prepared to pay, the social optimum is achieved only if the additional benefits are included. Thus, we need a mechanism to reveal the valuations of the free-riders.[5]

In the health field the main examples of pure public goods are drawn, not surprisingly, from public health measures. The eradication of malaria, for example, benefits all regardless of payment. Thus, in assessing the desirability of spending extensively to remove a disease, free-riders must somehow be taken into account.

2.3.3 Monopoly

The reader will already be aware that, in elementary theory, competition is preferred to monopoly because the monopolist devotes too few resources to his line of production as shown by the excess of price over marginal cost. This type of monopoly is usually described as 'unnatural' because it is a situation where a competitive industry could flourish. Monopoly power in this case arises for several reasons which could include sole ownership of a particular mineral right and patent laws giving one firm control over a particular industrial process. A monopoly may also occur because the local market that a particular firm supplies may be so small as to permit only one supplier. This would be a geographic or spatial monopoly. It is this latter case that might well apply in some instances to the health care field. A particular hospital or doctor may be the only one within acceptable travelling distance for a local community or communities, and as a consequence be the only source of supply of a commodity, namely health care, that has no close substitutes. This hospital is clearly in a position to make the monopoly profit that is the tribute profit-maximising monopolies levy on the consumers of their services and hence might be the target of government regulations.

There is a second type of monopoly, which can be seen as a more extreme case of the local monopoly, that may also be applied to the health care field. This is the natural monopoly, a situation where firms in an industry can achieve very considerable economies of scale, so much so that each fi[illegible] can meet the whole market level of demand alone without exhausting them. Economics of scale mean that long-run average cost (*AC*) and marginal cost (*MC*) decrease as output increases. Thus, if initially there are many firms in the industry, they each have an incentive to cut prices and expand sales as the extra output can be produced at a lower cost. However, if all firms act in this way, and assuming they cannot all attract extra sales, some firms will be forced out of business. This increases the sales of remaining firms and permits a further lowering of costs, again to the detriment of some firms. Ultimately only one firm remains. Such a monopoly is desirable as one firm can achieve lower production costs than many, but it raises other problems, shown in Figure 2.5. If it prices

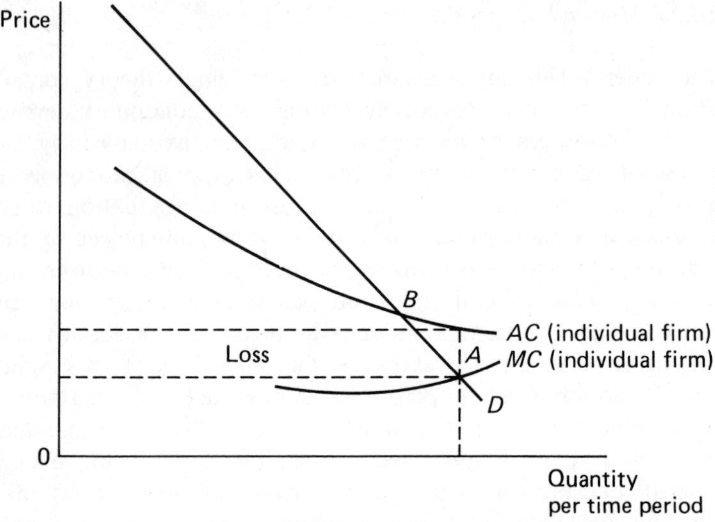

Figure 2.5 The hospital as a natural monopoly

above marginal cost, above *A* on the demand curve (*D*), or extracts monopoly profit at a price-quantity combination above *B* on the demand curve, then it distorts allocation at the margin. But optimal pricing at marginal cost leads to losses. The decreasing cost industry case (see for example Singer, 1976) is often applied to electricity generation, but it has been argued that hospitals may represent natural monopolies in that they can experience economies of scale or utilisation. This issue is discussed below in Chapter 7. For the moment we are content simply with the observation that monopoly elements may be found in the health care field and could be used as a case for some forms of government intervention to, say, concentrate activity in fewer hospitals and so achieve economies of scale, regulate fees charged, etc.

2.3.4 Uncertainty and choice

Lancaster (1966) has developed an approach to consumer choice based on the characteristics of goods. Consumers buy goods in order to enjoy these characteristics, be it relief of hunger by food or the relief of symptoms by health care. But while the consumer has a great deal of experience of the relationship between food and its ultimate effect on him, he has little or no knowledge of the correct health care to provide the characteristics he requires, e.g. relief from a disease or injury. Thus the doctor is in a peculiar position. Not only does he have more knowledge of the supply side of the market than the consumer, but also he has greater knowledge of the mix of services that it is appropriate for the consumer to demand.

The patient makes the initial decision to contact the doctor but typically allows the doctor to decide on his consumption of health care. Of course, budget constraints may prevent him from consuming the full package of services recommended, but, this aside, his effective choice is limited. (See Chapters 4 and 5 for a more detailed discussion of consumer demand and supplier-induced demand.) The doctors, for their part, exhibit the characteristics of most professions, one of which is not to criticise one's colleagues openly or to highlight failures, mistakes or instances of misconduct.[6] Regarding the quantity and type of care there is considerable variation in the therapies prescribed by different doctors, their duration and location for the same condition. The product of the health care sector is not the familiar homogeneous good of the perfect competition model. Entry to the profession is far from easy, there being considerable educational and licensing barriers to be overcome. Whatever the pros and cons of these characteristics, it seems clear that the consumer has little knowledge of the quality of care he receives and the cost of care. The importance of the latter is that if the price is overestimated too little medical care is chosen, and vice versa if it is underestimated. These uncertainties about the cost and quality of care, and indeed whether an identifiable illness will occur and is present or not, are highlighted by Arrow (1963), and are a recurring theme in this volume.

2.3.5 Merit wants

The concept of a merit want, introduced by Musgrave (1959), covers those private goods and services that are considered to be of such importance that they are financed and provided by the public sector in addition to the quantities produced and purchased in the market.

What is the rationale for the use of the merit want concept

in health care? Perhaps the most acceptable approach lies in questioning the information base on which consumers make choices about health care. The major issues discussed above related to uncertainty and the process of provision once contact is made. However, there are some additional considerations. First, people are ignorant of the presence of illness in some cases, or even if they are aware of illness they may be unaware of the consequences of not obtaining health care. Second, there are some instances where the imposed preferences implied by merit goods override the preferences of the individual. Some infringements on personal freedom may be acceptable even to the most ardent libertarian. These concern mental illness and unconscious emergency cases. In the former case society basically is saying that if an individual's behaviour or attitudes lie outside some arbitrary 'normal' range he forfeits the right to make choices for himself and has health care forced upon him. The latter case, although dramatic, is unlikely to be a very commonplace problem since the individual, if conscious, would typically agree to treatment. It is possible to interpret merit wants in other ways, but these tend to shade into externalities, e.g. as with the secondary poverty argument or into the 'enlightened despot' approach to the world where experts, or the more powerful, know what is best for society. The first instance is already under discussion and the second is inconsistent with the positive approach adopted in the chapters that follow. For a discussion of approaches to merit goods see Musgrave and Musgrave (1976).

2.4 More than one way to skin a cat

The major debate that took place in the early sixties relating to health economics concerned the policy relevance of the above characteristics. (For a convenient overview of the earlier exchanges see Lees *et al.*, 1964.) Even recently Lees has written 'The main question in the political economy of health services is the ancient one of the division of labour as between the individual and the state. What should be done voluntarily and in competitive markets and what collectively and compulsorily through government?' (Lees, 1976, p. 3). The two extremes were represented by those who felt, like Lees, that health care 'would appear to have no characteristics which differentiate it sharply from other goods in the market' (Lees, 1961, p. 21), and should, therefore, be dealt with in the market, and those who argued that health care was so different that government organisation and provision was appropriate (e.g. Titmuss, 1968). Culyer (1971) effectively ended the debate by arguing that the above characteristics could not be used to either prove or disprove the superiority of either form of provision, the question being essentially empirical. As a forerunner to the detailed theoretical discussions of the next chapter we review in brief here the strands of the debate on health care characteristics and policy. The possibilities are indicated below in the form of fencing match between Thrust and Parry.

Thrust: What about the externality problems of contagious diseases, primary and secondary poverty and option demand?

Parry: The contagious diseases or physical externality problem is of little practical significance, but in a market context this externality could be internalised by reducing the price of such inoculations (to OP_v^1 in Figure 2.3). Of course, providing immunisation free of user charge will also internalise the externality. In the above example it would lead to an extension of immunisation beyond the efficient level to OQ_v^2 but this is simply a result of the positions that have been given the supply and demand curves. A zero price or even a subsidy may be appropriate in the market.

The primary poverty argument is also relatively easily dealt with. It is very simply a question of redistributing income in favour of the poor. This could be achieved via a negative income tax, for example. The recipients of the additional income would then purchase health or more probably a health insurance policy, since deficient income is defined to be the cause of the problem. The secondary poverty case is more complex. It concerns individuals with sufficient income who do not, in the view of other individuals, spend a large enough proportion on health care. The way of eradicating the problem would seem to turn on its cause. If it is a question of the relevant individuals not being aware of the benefits of health care, then the subsidisation of information about health care would seem to be appropriate. This will not necessarily involve government provision of the information. If it is not an information problem, then the question becomes one of internalising an external cost imposed by those who do not value health care for themselves as highly as others do on their behalf. The methods by which externalities involved with health care can be internalised are discussed in detail in Chapter 3.

Solutions to the option demand problem (see Long, 1967; Lindsay, 1969) suggest that in a well-ordered insurance market there would be a wide range of insurance policies available. One variety would be a pre-payment policy whereby for a fixed sum in advance individuals are guaranteed all the health care they require in a coming time period. In these circumstances individuals would be able to opt into the prepayment policy that is associated with a hospital that maintains the 'correct' amount of excess capacity in the individual's view. However, it is also fair to say that a free, public system avoids the option demand problem by guaranteeing to treat the ill (after some delay, in less serious cases). Concern about the *physical* unavailability of treatment, should illness strike, is not common in Britain for this reason.

Thrust: This is all well and good, but surely you would agree that public goods problems require government intervention?

Parry: Certainly there is a case for intervention, but a role in the finance of public goods is sufficient. The spraying of the malarial swamp can be collectively financed via government without government provision. The same is also true of the public goods aspect of a generally felt externality.

Thrust: As well as recognising at least some role for government with public goods, you would surely agree that monopoly problems raise a similar case?

Parry: The pros and cons of monopoly are well rehearsed in the literature of economics. In this particular case relatively little has been said about hospitals as natural or unnatural monopolies. The position is complicated by the fact that private hospitals are often non-profit-making organisations. The answer to this worry of yours cannot be provided easily. (See Chapter 6 for a discussion of economic models of hospitals.)

Some have argued that an important problem with an extensive 'free' public system (e.g. the NHS) is that it denies individuals an 'exit voice'. In the market, suppliers competing with each other have an incentive to use their superior position to the consumers' advantage. Otherwise the individuals who are dissatisfied use their 'exit voice', leaving suppliers that do not provide a satisfactory service. However, it must be recognised that the Hippocratic oath may be a powerful check on doctors abusing their position, even if they do not face the normal restrictions of competition.

Thrust: Having essentially reserved your defense on monopoly, what about merit wants and the heading relating to information and uncertainty problems?

Parry: The mentally ill and the emergency patient seem to be conceded as cases requiring intervention though not necessarily by government. However, this argument can be applied only to a minority, leaving the majority to benefit from 'virtues' of the market mechanism. A relationship of trust between doctor and patient certainly would reduce the uncertainty problem that derives from the inequality of information, but as commentators have pointed out, is there any reason to believe that this relationship is better fostered in the public than in private sectors of the economy? As regards the uncertainty of the cost of care, public provision or private insurance remove this worry but at a price. Individuals face a tax bill or premium for their share of health care expenditure that is independent of their consumption. Thus, facing a zero price for care, consumers may demand a quantity of care that as tax- or premium-payers they are reluctant to supply.

It seems there are more answers than questions, and *a priori* it is impossible to decide whether a market-improving policy is superior to a market-displacing policy.

Finally, a point of agreement. Both Thrust and Parry agree that special policies would be required for the medically indigent who would find it difficult to purchase an insurance policy. The pro-market advocates, e.g. Lees, argue that to act as if special circumstances applied or should be applied to the whole of society is to throw out the baby with the bath water.

2.4.1 Has the point been missed?

One of the most vocal critics of an increasing role for the market in health care provision was the late Richard Titmuss. Although he attacked economists on their own ground in terms of the economic characteristics of health care (for example see Titmuss, 1968, Chapter 12, pp. 138–52), his fundamental criticism of the type of discussion given here is that an economic viewpoint cannot satisfactorily weigh up all the factors relating to health care provision. Titmuss's arguments (recently emphasised by Wilding, 1976) regarded social policy as being concerned with unilateral transfers (e.g. voluntary blood donation) and social integration. For Titmuss, health care provision was part of a broader social policy. Hence his view that 'the National Health Service in Britain has made a greater contribution to integration and ethnic tolerance than brigades of lawyers and platoons of social workers' (Titmuss *et al.*, 1968, p. 9). Titmuss emphasised the role and superiority of altruism in social relationships.

> Because (social policy) has continually to ask the question, 'who is my stranger?' it must inevitably be concerned with the unquantifiable and unmethodical aspects of man as well as with those aspects which can be identified and counted. Thus, in terms of policies, what unites it with ethical considerations is its focus on integrative systems: on processes, transactions and institutions which promote an individual's sense of identity, participation and community and allow him more freedom of choice for the expression of altruism and which, simultaneously, discourage a sense of individual alienation. [Titmuss, 1970, p. 224]

This much wider approach is beyond the scope of this study and, in our view, outside the economist's sphere. However, it does serve as a reminder that to some the issues discussed above do not represent an adequate conception of the debate over the appropriate roles of the market and the state in health care provision.

2.5 Summary

In this chapter three questions have been examined: Why do people seek health care? What are its main economic characteristics? What is the relevance of the latter for the provision of health care through private market or public non-market agencies? In response to the first question, health care as a source of pecuniary and non-pecuniary benefit was analysed. The economic characteristics of health care were considered under the headings that are usually used to question the desirability of the outcomes of the unaided market mechanism. In considering the third question, it was argued that the characteristics of health care made some form of government intervention essential in certain instances but that generally they did not imply the automatic superiority of market over non-market mechanisms or vice versa. Finally, the fact that it is specifically economic issues that have been discussed here was recognised, thereby hopefully avoiding the impression of economists presented by Titmuss, that they see themselves as 'possessively owning a hot line to God' (Titmuss, 1970; reprinted 1973, p. 225). Having introduced and reviewed some of the issues that affect the economic characteristics of health care, we now go on to consider in more detail the appropriateness of intervention by government when some subset of these characteristics is the focus for more detailed scrutiny.

NOTES

1. This is also shown by Grossman (1972), whose contribution is discussed in detail in Chapter 4.
2. These investment benefits are, in some of the literature on cost–benefit analysis, described as indirect benefits to distinguish them from the direct benefits described as reduced expenditure on health services in future time periods.
3. Strictly speaking, education can save lives, and some might argue that it saves more lives than health care. But it is normally viewed in the literature on the economics of education as increasing the productivity of the available work force. For a full discussion see Blaug (1970).
4. The possibility of economies of high wages via increased physical productivity because of better nutrition for those in employment is not discussed.
5. For a suggested solution to the free-rider problem see Groves and Loeb (1975).
6. For an early discussion of the economics of professions, see Lees (1966).

REFERENCES

Arrow, K. J. (1963) 'Uncertainty and the Welfare Economics of Medical Care', *American Economic Review*, Vol. 53, No. 5 (December), pp. 941–73; also reprinted as Reading 1 in Cooper and Culyer (1973).

BECKER, G. S. (1965) 'A Theory of the Allocation of Time', *Economic Journal*, Vol. 75, No. 299 (September), pp. 493–517.

BLAUG, M. (1970) *An Introduction to the Economics of Education*. Harmondsworth: Penguin.

COOPER, M. H. and CULYER, A. J. (eds.) (1973) *Health Economics*, Harmondsworth: Penguin.

CULYER, A. J. (1971) 'The Nature of the Commodity "Health Care" and its Efficient Allocation', *Oxford Economic Papers*, Vol. 23, No. 2 (July), pp. 189–211; excerpts from which are reprinted as Reading 2 in Cooper and Culyer (1973).

FUCHS, V. R. (1966) 'The Contribution of Health Services to the American Economy', *Milbank Memorial Fund Quarterly*, Vol. 44, Part 2 (October), pp. 65–101; reprinted as Chapter 1 in Fuchs, V. R. (ed.) (1972) *Essays in the Economics of Health and Medical Care*. New York and London: Columbia University Press for National Bureau of Economic Research.

GROSSMAN, M. (1972) *The Demand for Health: A Theoretical and Empirical Investigation*. (National Bureau of Economic Research Occasional Paper 119). New York and London: Columbia University Press.

GROVES, T. and LOEB, M. (1975) 'Incentives and Public Inputs', *Journal of Public Economics*, Vol. 4, pp. 211–26.

LANCASTER, K. (1966) 'A New Approach to Consumer Theory', *Journal of Political Economy*, Vol. 74, No. 2 (April), pp. 132–58.

LEES, D. S. (1960) 'The Economics of Health Services', *Lloyds Bank Review*, No. 56 (April), pp. 26–40.

LEES, D. S. (1961) *Health through Choice* (Hobart Paper No. 14). London: Institute of Economic Affairs; reprinted with additional material in *Freedom or Free-for-all? Essays in Welfare Trade and Choice*, Vol. 3 of the Hobart Papers (1965), pp. 21–93. London: Institute of Economic Affairs.

LEES, D. S. (1966) *Economic Consequences of the Professions* (Research Monograph 2). London: Institute of Economic Affairs.

LEES, D. S. (1976) 'Economics and Non-economics of Health Services', *Three Banks Review*, No. 110 (June), pp. 3–20.

LEES, D. S. *et al.* (1964) *Monopoly or Choice in Health Services* (Occasional Paper 3). London: Institute of Economic Affairs.

LINDSAY, C. M. (1969) 'Option Demand and Consumer's Surplus', *Quarterly Journal of Economics*, Vol. 83, No. 2 (May), pp. 344–6.

LONG, M. F. (1967) 'Collective-consumption Services of Individual-consumption Goods', *Quarterly Journal of Economics*, Vol. 81, No. 2 (May), pp. 351–2.

MINISTRY OF HEALTH (1956) *Report of the Committee of Enquiry into the cost of the NHS* (Guillebaud Report), Cmnd 9663. London: HMSO.

MUSGRAVE, R. A. (1959) *The Theory of Public Finance – A Study in Public Economy*. New York: McGraw-Hill.

MUSGRAVE, R. A. and MUSGRAVE P. B. (1976) *Public Finance in Theory and Practice*, 2nd edn. New York: McGraw-Hill.

MUSHKIN, S. J. (1962) 'Health as Investment', *Journal of Political Economy*, Vol. 70, No. 5(2), pp. 129–57; also reprinted as Reading 4 in Cooper and Culyer (1973).

PAGLIN, M. (1974) 'Public Health and Development, A New Analytical Framework', *Economica*, Vol. 41, No. 1 (November), pp. 432–41.

PESTON, M. (1972) *Public Goods and the Public Sector*. London and Basingstoke: Macmillan.

SINGER, N. M. (1976) *Public Microeconomics*, 2nd edn. Boston: Little, Brown.

TITMUSS, R. M. (1968) *Commitment to Welfare*. London: George Allen & Unwin.

TITMUSS, R. M. (1970) *The Gift Relationship – from Human Blood to Social Policy*. London: George Allen & Unwin; also published (1973): Harmondsworth: Penguin.

TITMUSS, R. M. *et al.* (1968) *Unequal Rights*. London: Child Poverty Action Group.

WEISBROD, B. A. (1964) 'Collective-consumption Services of Individual-consumption Goods', *Quarterly Journal of Economics*, Vol. 78, No. 3 (August), pp. 471–7.

WILDING, P. (1976) 'Richard Titmuss and Social Welfare', *Social and Economic Administration*, Vol. 10, No. 3 (Autumn), pp 147–66.

WISEMAN, J. (1963 'Cost-benefit Analysis and Health Service Policy', *Scottish Journal of Political Economy*, Vol. 10, No. 1 (February), pp. 128–45; also pp. 433–51 in Kiker, B. F. (ed.) (1971), *Investment in Human Capital*. Columbia, South Carolina: University of South Carolina Press.

WORLD BANK (1975) *Health* (Sector Policy Paper). Washington D.C.: World Bank.

3 Health Care and Market Intervention

> Medical care is a personal consumption good and as such is a dubious candidate for collective provision.
>
> *D. S. Lees* (1961, p. 21)

> This paper provides an economic explanation of the observed widespread support of direct public provision of medical care.
>
> *C. M. Lindsay* (1969, p. 531)

3.1 Introduction

In the last chapter we noted some of the reasons why health care does not conform to the theoretical characteristics of a good to be supplied by a market. In this chapter we examine in more detail a number of specific justifications for intervention in the market for health care. These concern two aspects. The first involves the importance of health and health care as sources of interpersonal utility dependence; i.e., the consumption of health care by one individual affects the utility of another. The second involves the effects of uncertainty and the problems that arise when the market alone provides insurance cover for health care expenditures.

3.2 Interdependent preferences

In the elementary theory of consumers' choice it is explicitly assumed that individual preference functions are independent of each other. That is, Mr A's utility is derived from his consumption of goods 1, 2, 3, 4, ... n and is independent of the levels of consumption of these goods by Mr B., so that the two individuals utility functions would be represented as:

$$U_A = U_A(X_A^1, X_A^2, X_A^3, \ldots, X_A^n)$$

$$U_B = U_B(X_B^1, X_B^2, X_B^3, \ldots, X_B^n).$$

As indicated in Chapter 2 above, much of the literature relating to health care departs from this assumption and assumes that individuals have the health care of others as an argument in their utility function. However, the implications that follow depend on the precise form of interdependence assumed. We consider below the implications of three variations on this theme for government intervention in the market for health care before turning to a further set of issues thrown up by uncertainty and insurance.

3.2.1 Sharing and a national health service

Lindsay (1969) postulates a society in which there 'may be a universal desire and willingness to share' (p. 531). He argues that, in an egalitarian society with individuals demonstrating the same medical need (an assumption of the model), what is desired is more equal treatment. The typical member of an S-person society has a utility function depicted as follows:

$$U_j = U_j(X_j^1, X_j^2, \ldots, X_j^n, h_j, e)$$

where X_j^i $(i = 1, \ldots, n)$ are the quantities of n goods consumed by the jth. individual, h_j is his consumption of health care and e is a measure of the distribution of health care consumption about its mean, $\bar{h}$.

$$e = -\sum_{j=1}^{S} |\bar{h} - h_j|$$

so that the individual's utility level is a function not only of the goods and services he consumes $(X_j^1, X_j^2, \ldots, X_j^n, h_j)$ but also the degree of equality with which health care is distributed. Any deviation of an individual's consumption of health care from the mean h exerts a negative influence on the utility of *each and every* member of a society. Lindsay developed the model using simple supply and demand analysis and a two-person society. Assume a rich individual, A, whose demand for health care,

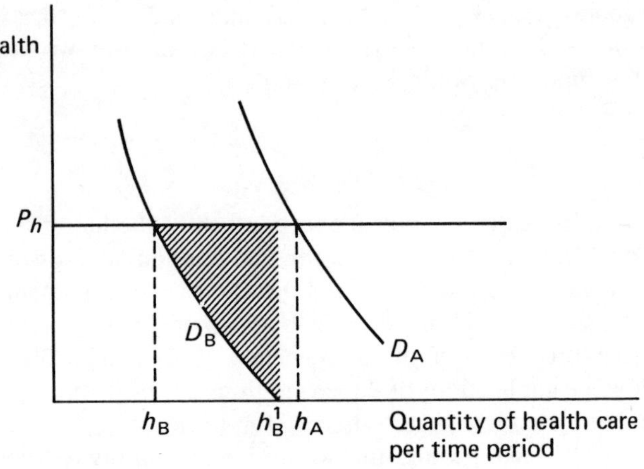

Figure 3.1 A's and B's demand for health care

a normal good, can be represented by D_A and a poor person, B, whose demand can be represented by D_B. In Figure 3.1 what is valued is a reduction in the difference between the two individuals' optimum private purchases, h_A, h_B, given the perfectly elastic supply curve for health care at price P_h. If the assumption of a two-person society is dropped, the 'free-rider' problem raises its ugly head. Any unilateral activity to promote greater equality provides a positive externality to all other members of this concerned society. Hence, it is only collective action that will extend the equality-promoting activity to its optimum extent. The free-rider problem and the need for collective action also become issues in the Culyer model discussed below once the simplifying assumption of a two-person society is relaxed. To determine the appropriate nature of intervention, the costs of different methods and, more important, the costs of sharing have to be considered. The four possibilities are illustrated in Figure 3.2.

The first, the burnt offering method (*BO*) means individual A purchasing his optimum quantity of health care, h_A, but simply consuming nearer h_B, i.e. throwing away some proportion of h_A. The cost curve associated with this option is P_hBO. The first or marginal unit thrown away is valued at OP_h, the market price. However, the second and subsequent units are valued more highly to the extent of individual A's consumer surplus from purchasing health care, so that the cost of the burnt offering

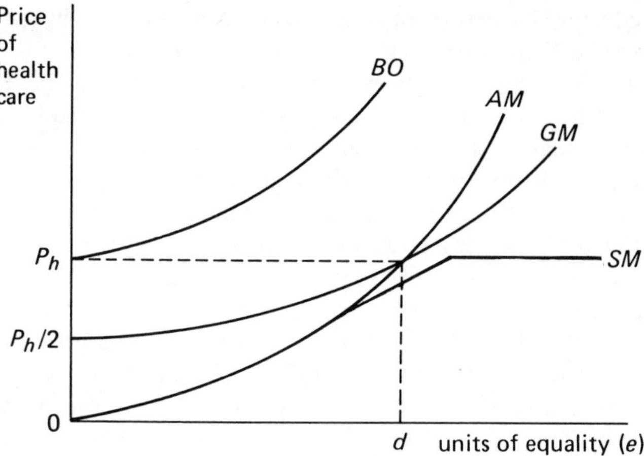

Figure 3.2 The costs of sharing

method is simply that portion of A's demand curve above OP_h, laterally reflected.

The gift method (*GM*), intuitively much more sensible, involves purchasing at h_A but giving units of health care to B so that his consumption of medical care is extended beyond h_B at one and the same time as A's is reduced below h_A, a double incursion on inequality. This reduces inequality at half the cost per unit of the *BO* method. The cost curve of *GM* is thus $P_h/2GM$, a curve with a slope equal to half $P_h BO$ and an intercept of half the cost of P_h.

The third method (*AM*) involves A buying a lower quantity of health care than his optimum. This only produces equality in the same one-for-one ratio as (*BO*) but has the advantage that it involves no monetary outlay by A as his sacrifice is simply his consumer surplus loss from not buying his optimum quantity of medical care, i.e. *OAM*.

Finally, there is the subsidy method (*SM*). Here we are concerned with the cost of inducing B to purchase more units of health care. The maximum a one-unit increase in the equality of health care can cost is P_h when A meets the whole cost per unit. Earlier units, those between h_B and h_B^1 in Figure 3.1, however, should cost less than this because A could offer to bear that portion of the price of marginal units that exceeds B's marginal valuation of them, i.e. the shaded area above D_B in Figure 3.1. The cost of reducing inequality of health care consumption by subsidy method is, therefore, *OSM*.

Since it is not possible to offer the same unit to be burnt, given or not bought, a choice of methods has to be made. Note, however, that it is possible to combine any *one* of these three methods with the subsidy method, thereby producing an overall cost-of-sharing curve that is the horizontal sum of the subsidy method and the least cost of the other three methods. *BO* is everywhere more expensive than the other methods and can, therefore, be ignored. *SM* is cheaper than the others at all levels and can, therefore always be used. However, as discussed above, *SM* can be combined with *AM* or *GM*. Which one will be chosen? Looking at Figure 3.2 and ignoring *SM* for the moment, it can be seen that below *Od*, *AM* is the least-cost method whereas above *Od*, *GM* is the least-cost method. Now the maximum cost of a unit of equality generated via the subsidy method is P_h, and therefore the method that is least-cost below P_h is the one to combine with *SM*. As it turns out, the cross-over point where *AM* ceases to be less costly compared with *GM* occurs at price level P_h so that over the relevant range *AM* is superior to *GM*, and it is therefore *AM* that should be horizontally summed with *SM* to give the least overall cost curve for generating units of equality. That the cross-over point of *AM* and *GM* occurs at P_h can be seen as follows:

$$BO = 2GM \tag{3.1}$$

$$BO = AM + P_h. \tag{3.2}$$

Substituting for *BO* in (3.1),

$$AM + P_h = 2GM \tag{3.3}$$

$$\therefore AM = 2GM - P_h. \tag{3.4}$$

At the intersection

$$AM = GM. \tag{3.5}$$

Hence

$$AM - GM = GM - P_h = 0. \tag{3.6}$$

Therefore

$$AM = GM = P_h. \tag{3.7}$$

To recap, the subsidy method is the least-cost way of producing units of equality. However, because subsidising B and either 'giving' or 'burning' or 'abstaining' on A's part are not mutually exclusive events, the overall least-cost curve is the horizontal sum of the subsidy method and one other. The least-cost method of the other three over the relevant range below P_h has been shown to be the abstention method, *AM*; hence it is chosen to be combined with the subsidy method, *SM*. In Figure 3.3 *AM* and *SM* are the cost-of-sharing curves facing the individual voters and *OdfSM* is the horizontal sum of the two. If the voters' demand for equality is D_e the optimum quantity is *Og*, and the appropriate policy is *Oa* of abstention or rationing, and *Os* of subsidy. This, argues Lindsay, is the NHS where the subsidy method corresponds to finance via progressive taxation and the abstention method corresponds to the requirement that the NHS administers equally to all.

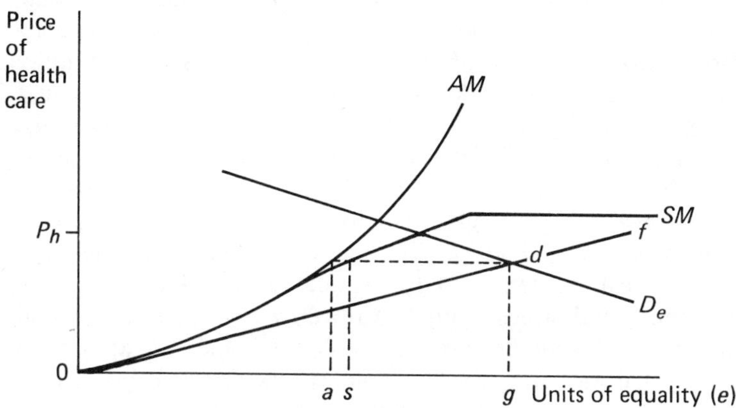

Figure 3.3 Lindsay's NHS

3.2.2 Giving and a national health service

Culyer (1971) has attempted to establish the view that it is the *quantity* of suffering felt by individuals rather than its distribution over individuals that forms the basis of the externality relationships that predict an NHS-type organisation. Using one rich individual

(A) and one poor individual (B), we can redefine their utility functions as follows:

$$U_A = U_A(X_A{}^1, X_A{}^2, \ldots, X_A{}^n, h_A, h_B)$$
$$U_B = U_B(X_B{}^1, X_B{}^2, \ldots, X_B{}^n, h_B)$$

A has what is known as a *specifically interdependent* utility function (See Hochman and Rodgers, 1969). In simple terms, A's utility is dependent not only on the goods and services he consumes, but the *quantity* of one specific good, health care (h), that individual B consumes. The analysis uses a triangular Edgeworth–Bowley trading box. This construction differs from the normal Edgeworth–Bowley trading box in that on the x-axis is B's health care and any given quantity of it is a source of utility for *both* A and B. In the normal rectangular trading box the good on the x-axis has no public good characteristics and any given quantity of good or service along it is a source of utility for either A or B only.

The triangular Edgeworth–Bowley trading box then enables the analysis of a private good and what is in effect here a public good. (N.B. It is the health care itself that is the source of utility for B whereas it is the knowledge that B has health care that is the source of utility to A and all individuals who think like him in society – it is the latter that has the public good characteristics.) The triangular trading box is constructed as follows. Y is the *numeraire* commodity which for simplicity can be interpreted as income. O_A and O_B are A and B's respective origins, and their vertical separation in Figure 3.5 represents the extent of community endowment with Y, with $O_A Y$ and $O_B Y$ their initial allocations. A's indifference curves, $I_A{}^0$, $I_A{}^1$ and $I_A{}^2$, are drawn in the usual way, with a negative slope indicating that his endowment of the *numeraire* commodity and the quantity of B's health care are both 'goods' to him. B's indifference curves have been squeezed up to fit in the triangular box in the following manner. Figure 3.4(a) represents the initial position for B with equilibrium occuring at point (β) permitting utility level $I_B{}^0$. The slope of Yg (and $I_B{}^0$ at β) represents the rate at which B can substitute income for health care (as with the normal budget line).

The slope of the h_B axis and B's indifference curve is now increased by a constant equal to the rate at which society can convert income into B's medical care.[1] The effect of this is to

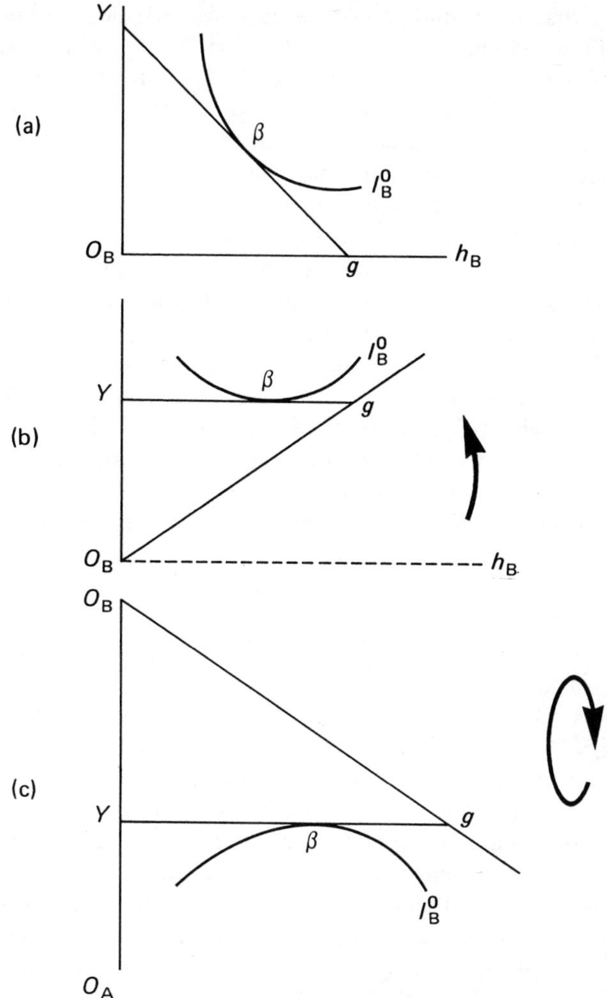

Figure 3.4 Constructing the triangular Edgeworth–Bowley trading box

squeeze up Figure 3.4(a) to form Figure 3.4(b). The final step is to invert B's 'adjusted' indifference map and place it on A's so that the distance $O_A O_B$ measures the sum of A's and B's initial endowment of Y (i.e. $O_A O_B = O_A Y + O_B Y$). A numerical example may make this process more clear. Suppose the slope of Yg in Figure 3.4(a) is (−) 3 : 1; i.e., 3 units of income must be sacrificed for 1 unit of health care. If we add to this and the indifference curve $I_B{}^0$ a constant equal to this ratio (i.e. the slope of Yg and $I_B{}^0$ at β), then the slope of Yg and $I_B{}^0$ at β becomes zero i.e. a horizontal straight line as in Figure 3.4(b). The slopes of all B's indifference curves are no longer his marginal rate of substitution between health care and income but rather the difference between his marginal rate of substitution and marginal rate of transformation between income and health care.[2]

In Figure 3.5 O_Bv represents all possible combinations of Y and B's medical care that are available to this two-person society. Given his endowment of income, O_BY, it can be seen that B, left to his own devices, will adjust to position β on his highest attainable utility curve $I_B{}^0$. A, on the other hand, can adjust individually along Yt. However, B's purchase of O_Ar of health care has the effect of pushing out A's consumption possibilities to $Y\beta u$, since for any given purchase of care for B by A, B's consumption is higher by an amount $O_Ar(= Y\beta = tu)$. B's purchase

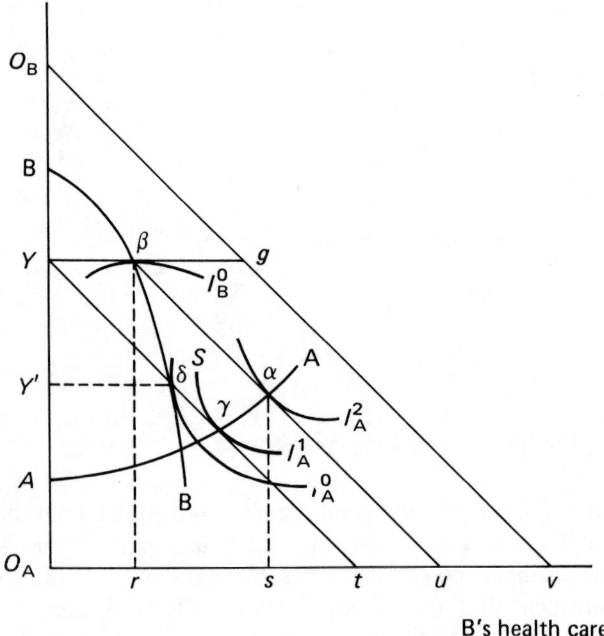

Figure 3.5 Culyer's NHS

of health care is in effect a lump-sum spill-in to A (see Williams, 1966). With B buying $Y\beta(=tu)$ health care, A's highest attainable utility level occurs at α on $I_A{}^2$. This involves A in buying *rs* of health care for B (remember the level of B's health care consumption is a source of utility for A). This, however, implies that A prefers a level of consumption of health care by B above B's optimum level $Y\beta(=O_Ar)$, and hence B will cease to buy health care for himself allowing A to buy all his health care on his behalf. A's highest attainable utility level if B ceases to buy health care is at γ on $I_A{}^1$. This is philanthropy-in-kind.

Culyer compares philanthropy-in-kind, the NHS approach, with philanthropy-in-money. In the latter case the effect will be to displace downwards what is in effect B's budget line *Yg* by the amount of the income transfer. For each income transfer he receives, B chooses a quantity of health care that maximises his utility. The locus of these points of equilibrium under income transfers is *BB*; i.e., *BB* is a consumption income expansion path. (Analogously, *AA* is the expansion path for A's purchased care for B when his income is not transferred to B.) A, who can dictate this process of income transfer, will choose the transfer that maximises his utility level. This is point δ on indifference curve $I_A{}^0$ (where $I_A{}^0$ tangents to *BB*). Achieving $I_A{}^0$ involves transferring YY' of income to B. A in this construction prefers philanthropy-in-kind, as this yields him a higher level of utility (at γ) than philanthropy-in-money (at δ). Note that B also prefers philanthropy-in-kind and so both rich and poor will vote for a NHS. However, this result of both A and B preferring an NHS-type organisation does depend on the shape of the indifference maps attributed to A and B, and so legitimates intervention by provision-in-kind as a special case and not a generally valid result.

3.2.3 Externalities and insurance

Pauly (1971) adopted a similar interdependent utility framework in examining optimal health care consumption. The model requires the following assumptions: health care consumption generates marginally relevant externalities; health care is produced and sold at a constant marginal cost; health care has a positive income elasticity; any individual's marginal evaluation of care for his fellow members of society is independent of his own consumption level; there is no strategic bargaining; preferences are expressed efficiently; and all individuals have identical utility functions relating to their own consumption of health care (which implies that observed consumption differences are simply a consequence of income differences). In Figure 3.6 *MC* is the constant marginal cost curve, D_A, D_B and D_C are the demand curves for three persons, of whom individual C has the lowest income and individual A the highest. D_S is the social marginal evaluation curve for care and is made up of the aggregate of the three individuals' marginal evaluation curves for health care for every one in the community excluding themselves. ΣD_A, ΣD_B and ΣD_C are the vertical summations of the individual (internal) and society's (external) marginal evaluations for the three individuals. Given these circumstances, optimal consumption levels are h_A^*, h_B^* and h_C^* for individuals A, B and C respectively. (N.B. Individual A, left to his own devices, will consume more than enough health care in the eyes of the remainder of the community.) However, the policy problem is that individuals B and C will equate their own demand and supply curves and consume inefficiently low quantities of health care at h_B and h_C respectively. What is the appropriate mechanism to raise their consumption levels? Pauly considered several possibilities. The force of the law could be used so that B and C would be legally required to consume h_B^* and h_C^* units

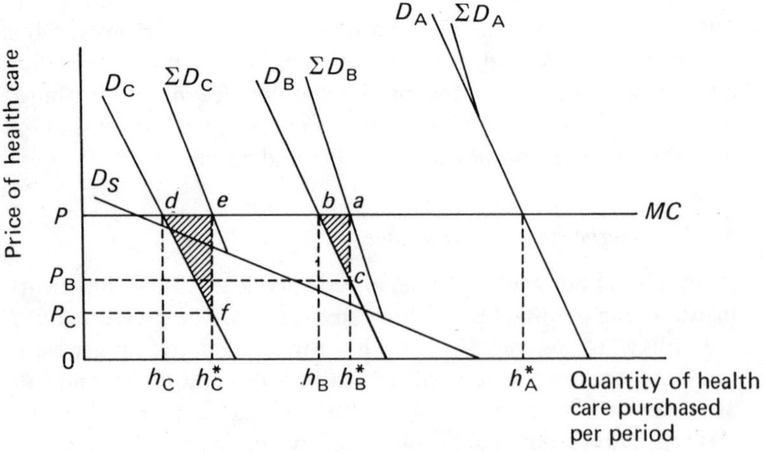

Figure 3.6 Pauly's optimal insurance scheme

of health care. However, the burden of this policy falls heaviest on the poorest individual. For B the cost of the additional units of health care is area $h_B h_B{}^*ab$ but benefits amount only to area $h_B h_B{}^*c$, b and so he suffers an efficiency loss to the extent of the shaded triangle (abc). For C the respective magnitudes are $h_C h_C{}^*d$, e and $h_C h_C{}^*fd$, giving an efficiency loss of $(def) > (abc)$, clearly an inequitable policy. Free, but limited, care is an alternative policy. But this is likely to have little impact in extending the consumption of health care because of the considerable likelihood that, faced with free public care, individuals would cease to purchase health care of their own account. One alternative solution involves using prices to extend health care consumption. Using subsidies, the effective prices of health care to individuals could be adjusted downwards to P_C for individual C and P_B for individual B and remain at P for individual A. This would induce the efficient consumption of health care by all three but would require subsidies based on individuals' own demand and not an administratively simpler general subsidy.

3.3 Risk aversion and risk preference

We now turn to one further aspect of health care on which policy recommendations have been based, the uncertainty of ill health occurring and the scope for insurance. However, since insurance is simply protection against risk, we examine first the characteristics of risk averse consumers. (A full exposition can be found in Green, 1976.)

Suppose an individual with a positive marginal utility of wealth is faced with a choice between a certain amount of wealth, say £1000, and a 50–50 chance of £800 or £1200, the actual outcome being determined by the toss of a fair coin. Since $\frac{1}{2}$(£800) + $\frac{1}{2}$(1200) = £1000, the expected outcome matches the certain outcome and so is described as a fair bet (i.e., in the long run, anyone staking £1000 on a series of such bets would expect to break even). Risk-averters reject a single fair bet because of their preference for certainty, whereas risk-preferers accept one. Assuming we know the utility associated with sums of £800 and £1200, we can plot them as points F and G in Figure 3.7. The

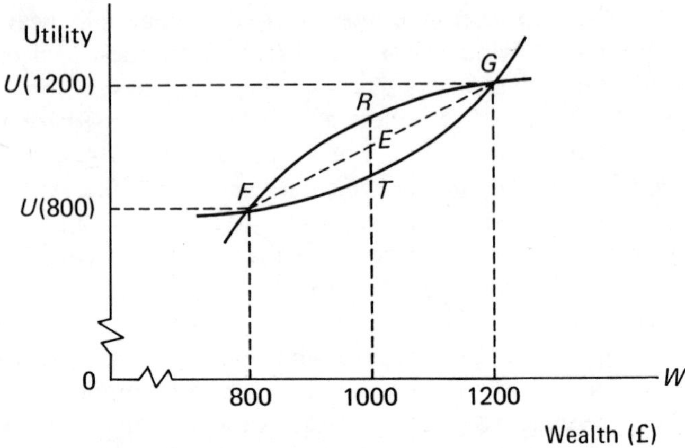

Figure 3.7 Risk and the marginal utility of wealth

expected utility associated with accepting the bet can then be found by plotting the utility level associated with the expected outcome $\frac{1}{2}U(£800) + \frac{1}{2}U(£1200)$, i.e., E (a point midway between $W = £800$ and $W = £1200$ on a straight line between F and G. If an individual accepts the uncertain outcome of either £800 or £1200, then the utility of £1000 is at a point like T below E. He prefers $\frac{1}{2}U(£800) + \frac{1}{2}U(£1200)$ to $U(£1000)$ and is a risk-preferer. If the individual rejects the bet, then $U(£1000)$ is above E at say, R. Joining *FRG* and *FTG* it can be seen that an increasing marginal utility of wealth (i.e. increasing slope of the utility function) is equivalent to risk preference and decreasing marginal utility of wealth is the equivalent of risk aversion.

3.3.1 Will individuals insure against health care expenses?

Assume an individual has diminishing marginal utility of wealth. Then his utility function could look like the curve (*AA*) in Figure 3.8(a2). Now suppose over a given period this individual has the choice of insuring against medical care expenses at a fair premium or choosing to be uninsured and cover out of his pocket any health care expenses he incurs; what will he choose to do? If he is risk-*averse* as discussed above and indicated by the utility of wealth functions, he will choose to take out insurance, whereas if he is a risk-taker he will assume the risk of incurring expenses

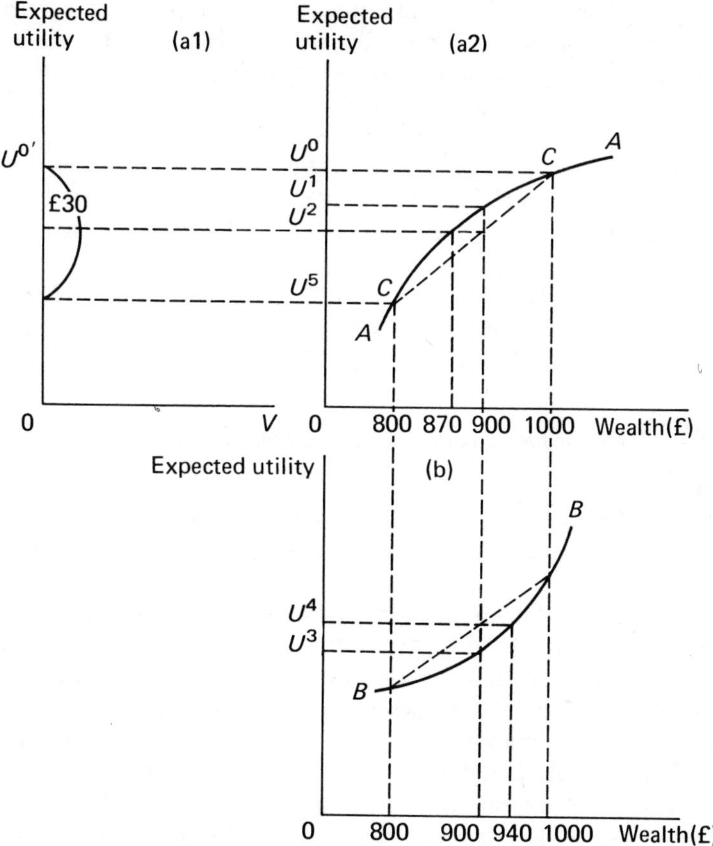

Figure 3.8 (a1) the value of the service of insurance (V); (a2) the risk-averter; (b) the risk-taker

himself. Let us assume that the premium is £100 per time period, the probability that he will require treatment is 0.5, and his income is £1000 (i.e., he is insured against £200 of medical care expenses). The individual will now face a situation where he can have a certain income of £900 and health care insurance or 0.5 chance of £1000 and a similar chance of £800. The expected utility of the former is OU^1 and of the latter OU^2; i.e., the utility level associated with $0.5 \times £800 + 0.5 \times £1000$ (the utility level associated with a point halfway along the dashed line *CC*). Hence our individual prefers to be insured. Indeed, he would be prepared to pay as much as £30 in addition to the fair premium charge in order to be insured. A probabilistic £900 has the same utility level, OU^2, associated with it as a 'certain' £870.

However, if our individual has increasing marginal utility of wealth/income the position is as in Figure 3.8(b). Here the individual enjoys utility level OU^3 with insurance and OU^4, a higher utility level, without. Indeed, the risk-taker will be prepared to pay a sum equal to say £40 in order to avoid having to buy insurance; i.e. a probabilistic £900 has the same utility level, OU^4, associated with it as a certain £940. Returning to our original question, it can be seen that risk averters prefer to insure against health care expenses.

3.3.2 The case for compulsory government insurance

The implications of behaviour towards risk for health care provision have been developed by Arrow (1963), in one of the key articles in the literature. 'The special economic problems of medical care can be explained as adaptations to the existence of uncertainty in the incidence of disease and in the efficacy of treatment' (Arrow, 1963, p. 941). Specifically Arrow stressed two types of risk: 'the risk of becoming ill and the risk of total or incomplete or delayed recovery' (p. 959) and argues that 'from the point of view of the welfare economics of uncertainty, both losses are risks against which individuals would like to insure. The non-existence of suitable insurance policies for either risk implies a loss of welfare' (p. 959). Arrow has also compared the operation of the medical care market with perfect competition under conditions of certainty and uncertainty. It is in this last section that he attempts to demonstrate that the characteristics of health care can be explained 'either as the result of deviations from the competitive preconditions or as attempts to compensate by other institutions for these failures' (p. 948).

The characteristics considered by Arrow should be familiar to the reader by now. They comprise the irregular and unpredictable nature of demand and the high cost in terms of lost productive capacity that the individual might incur should illness strike; the behaviour of the physician, who is expected not to advertise or price-compete, to ignore his own self-interest when treating patients, to divorce treatment from any financial considerations, and to be objective in the provision of information, e.g. in certifying illness; the uncertainty as to the quality of the product, uncertainty of recovery, the inability to 'shop around', and the super production and consumption knowledge of the doctor. The restriction of entry by licensing, the minor share of the cost of medical education borne by the student and limited places at medical school are noted under the heading of supply conditions.

Four particular aspects receive attention in the comparison of medical care with the competitive norm. First, the general interdependence that can be found in the health care field is emphasised, i.e. 'the concern of individuals for the health of others' (Arrow, 1963, p. 954). Second, the possibility of increasing returns playing some role is noted. Thirdly, the entry restrictions mentioned above are discussed more fully and the effects of entry restrictions excluding imperfect substitutes for physicians is expanded upon. Finally the pricing issue is discussed, especially in relation to Kessel's (1958) argument that price discrimination is an attempt by the medical profession to use their monopoly power to maximise profits. The fourth section compares the actual operation of the medical care market with a world in which insurance policies against all conceivable risks are available.

Having discussed the theory of ideal insurance, Arrow argued that 'the welfare case for insurance policies of all sorts is overwhelming. It follows that the government should undertake insurance in those cases where the market, for whatever reason, has failed to emerge' (Arrow, 1963, p. 961). Arrow recognised some of the problems involved with insurance but concluded that they do not 'alter the case for the creation of a much wider class of insurance policies than now exists' (p. 961).

However, a number of arguments have been proposed to explain why even risk-averters may not buy insurance. (N.B. We know risk-lovers will choose not to buy health care insurance.) These focus on the transactions costs and the demand elasticity of medical care, both of which affect insurance. Lees and Rice (1965) took issue with Arrow for ignoring buyers' and sellers' costs and hence assuming that fair insurance is available. Account needs to be taken of administration and the other selling expenses, as well as of the time, trouble and money costs of an insurance policy. Using Figure 3.8(a1), the amount (V) that an individual is prepared to pay in excess of the fair premium for £200 worth of insurance is indicated by the half-moon shape $U^{0\prime}U^{5\prime}$ for all the probabilities of the insurance being required, i.e. those between 0 and 1. Fair insurance F can be defined (as it has implicitly been above) as the premium determined by multiplying the probability P that the event to be insured against will occur and the number N and cost C of units of health care to be provided in that event: $F = P(NC)$. It is clear in Figure 3.8(a1) that the more certain or more uncertain the event is, the less is the individual prepared to pay the sum over and above the fair premium (i.e., when the event is very likely or very unlikely to occur, the advantage of having insurance is less). Now assume, with Lees and Rice, that the cost of insurance services (CI) varies with the fair premium in constant proportional relationships; i.e., $CI = kP(NC)$. The smaller the probability of a given (NC), the greater the likelihood that the excess the individual is prepared to pay over the fair premium is greater than CI and the more likely that insurance coverage will be observed. This is illustrated in Figure 3.9.

Below $p(nc)$ the value the individual places on being insured over and above the fair premium is greater than Cl and insurance is observed for a given NC. Given transactions cost, not all medical expenditures will be insured against. Arrow's (1965) reply to this line of criticism was partly one of surprise that the explicit recognition of the costs of (privately) marketing insurance by Lees and Rice was used as an argument against alternative methods of resource allocation. After discussing transactions costs and differ-

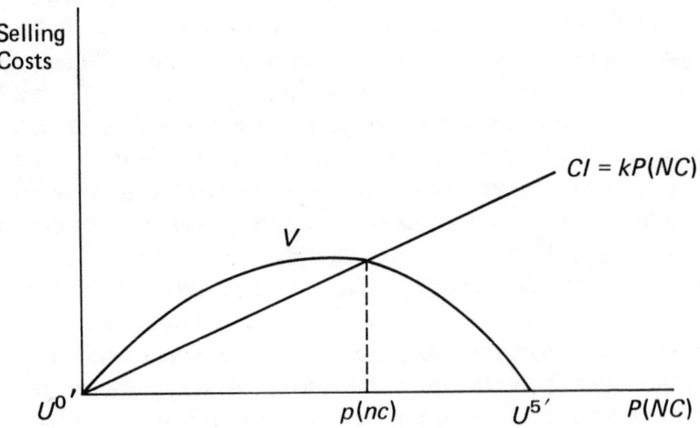

Figure 3.9 The value of the service of insurance (V) and selling costs

ent modes of economic organisation, seeing the former reduced under a government universal insurance scheme, Arrow concluded that

> Clearly, further innovation is desirable in the provision of health insurance, and I see no convincing argument that, in the absence of alternatives, it is undesirable or unnecessary for it to take the form of an increased role for the government. [Arrow, 1965, p. 157–8]

This is an important issue that is reopened in Chapter 11.

Pauly (1968) has offered a different explanation of why some insurances are not offered commercially. He argues that only if demand is perfectly inelastic with respect to price in the range from market prices to zero is a health care or other expense insurable in the sense envisaged by Arrow. Pauly's argument relies on the notion of moral hazard. The latter is a problem associated with insurance systems. Fair insurance (F) was defined above as: $F = P(NC)$. The problem is that once people have knowledge that they are insured their behaviour can be altered in two ways. First, the probability that the event will occur may increase. Individuals insured against health care expenses may well be careless with their health, increasing P to P'. Second, once the event occurs individuals may well demand a quality or quantity of health care that exceeds the original sum to be covered, i.e. increasing N to N'. The *ex ante* fair insurance sum is thus too small a premium for the *ex post* position $P'.N'.C$.

Pauly based his argument only on the latter of these possibilities, the increase in the total amount of care demanded once insurance has been taken up and the event occurs. A simple example will illustrate his argument. Suppose in a given period an individual faces a half chance of keeping well and not requiring health care and a half chance of being ill and requiring 100 units of health care. Assuming health care is supplied along a perfectly elastic supply curve at the price £5 per unit, then the fair insurance premium equals

$$£250 = \tfrac{1}{2} \,.\, 0 \,.\, £5 + \tfrac{1}{2} \,.\, 100 \,.\, £5.$$

The situation is illustrated in Figure 3.10, where demand for health care D_A is initially assumed to be inelastic and coincides with the y-axis in the event that individual A remains well. Should the individual become ill, D_A' is the relevant demand curve, being

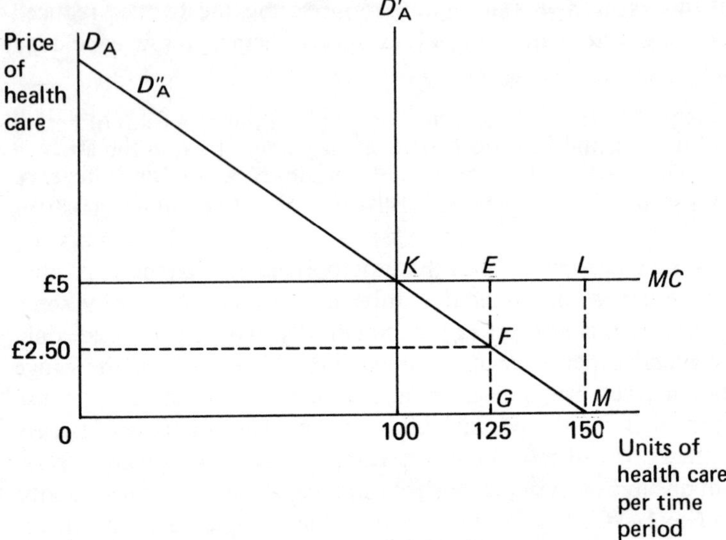

Figure 3.10 Moral hazard and insurance

perfectly inelastic at 100 units of health care. In this case the *ex ante* and *ex post* fair premium are identical. The moral hazard problem arises once the demand curve for health care exhibits a degree of elasticity as with demand curve D_A''. Now, once illness strikes, the individual demands 150 units of health care, paid for by his insurers. Once his behaviour with insurance is taken account of a fair premium becomes:

$$£375 = \tfrac{1}{2} . 0 . £5 + \tfrac{1}{2} . 150 . £5.$$

The individual may not choose to accept insurance at the fair premium his behaviour, once insured, dictates, namely £375. His decision will depend upon whether the efficiency loss that arises on the last 50 units of care consumed with insurance is more or less than the utility gain that arises from being insured, i.e. the amount this individual would be prepared to pay for the *service* of insurance (represented as *V* above). In this case *V* would have to exceed *KLM* or £125 = (50 . £2.50). This may well not be the case. The inference is that risk-averse individuals, when faced with premiums that take account of moral hazard, may well reject insurance against medical care expenses. But although individuals reject full insurance they might accept another form of insurance. There are devices that can be introduced into insurance policies that can help overcome the moral hazard problem. A deductible is one possibility. Here the individual if ill has to pay for the first specified number of units at the market price, the remainder being free of charge. In our example 125 units is the deductible that is marginal. This is because the efficiency or consumer surplus loss, incurred because the units paid for between 100 and 125 at the market price exceed their marginal value to the extent of *KEF*, is exactly balanced by the consumer surplus gain accruing to the 'free' units of health care between 125 and 150, i.e. *FGM*. For a deductible below 125 the individual will accept the insurance policy, whereas he will reject one above 125. In the former case the deductible has no impact on the quantity of health care consumed in the event of illness, namely 150 units. If the deductible is rejected then the quantity of health care consumed in the event of illness becomes the no-insurance level of 100 units.

A second device is co-insurance. Here the insured individual has to pay a certain proportion of each unit of health care consumed in the case of illness. In Figure 3.10, for a co-payment of 50 per cent, £2.50 per unit has to be paid by the individual, reducing the quantity of medical care demanded to 125 units. Other insurance schemes include fixed indemnity, where the individual is insured for a given expenditure on health care and prepayment, where for some fixed sum in advance the individual is covered for all the health care he may require in the period covered. The literature also makes mention of self-insurance. The latter simply means the assumption of one's own risk. In these circumstances individuals can act to reduce the probability of ill health, e.g. by taking care crossing roads, and can reduce expenditures should illness strike by maintaining the recuperative capacity of the body, say through a sensible diet. Insurance is discussed further below, especially in Chapter 11. The point of emphasis here is that Arrow was wrong in assuming that the presence of uninsured risk-averse people automatically implied market failure.

Arrow (1968), in reply to Pauly, accepts that the latter shows that 'the optimality of complete insurance is no longer valid when the method of insurance influences the demand for the services provided by the insurance policy' (Arrow, 1968, p. 537).

However, he goes on to argue that non-market controls could be introduced to ration the amount of health care to the insurance-supported quantity and thus avoid or minimise the moral hazard problem. The possibilities cited are: (a) insurance company monitoring of items provided, (b) reliance on physicians not to prescribe frivolously, and (c) reliance on the individual to behave in line with some commonly accepted norms and self-restraint.

3.4 Summary

This chapter has looked at two broad issues: the implications of interdependent utility functions for the form of health care provision, and the issue of (government-provided) insurance for health care. Regarding the former, the models presented are elegant and interesting within themselves. In addition, Lindsay and Pauly show how considerable implications can be drawn from imaginative use of only the simplest tools of economic analysis – supply and demand. As regards Lindsay and Culyer, the latter model can be preferred on the grounds that it is more simple in terms of the externality relationship it postulates. But as Culyer himself points out, neither model explains the key feature of the UK NHS, that is its presence in the public sector. If the concern is with increasing the consumption of health care, why are price reductions not adopted as in the Pauly model? This major weakness of the NHS 'explanations' indicates that the socio-political context in which the NHS was set is of fundamental importance to a full understanding of the genesis of the NHS.

On the question of insurance, Arrow's exposition of the problems is central. We have concentrated here on the particular issues of moral hazard and transaction costs because of their theoretical importance, but neither is wholly resolved in the theoretical literature. In addition, there are a number of practical dimensions of insurance provision that present similar problems. These will be held over until our review of health care provision in the United States (Chapter 11).

For the present, we can note the models of this chapter as attempts to build a theoretical case for intervention in the market that are not wholly successful but highlight a number of significant facets of the topic. Having come this far in considering general issues of market organisation, we now turn to the microeconomics of demand and supply since these have some further implications for the pricing and organisation of health care services.

NOTES

1. If the initial transformation curve is of the form, $Y = \overline{Y} - k.h$, with slope of $-K$, adding Kh to this transformation curve gives $Y = \overline{Y} - K.h + K.h = Y$, a horizontal line. Similarly, adding Kh to the h axis shifts it to Kh. All the indifference curves are similarly shifted by the addition of Kh, i.e. an increase in slope of $+K$.
2. If this construction is still not clear see Dolbear (1967) and Shibata (1971).

REFERENCES

ARROW, K. J. (1963) 'Uncertainty and the Welfare Economics of Medical Care', *American Economic Review*, Vol. 53, No. 5 (December), pp. 941–73; also reprinted as reading 1 in Cooper and Culyer (1973).

ARROW, K. J. (1965) 'Reply' ('The Implications of Transactions Costs and Adjustment Lags'), *American Economic Review*, Vol. 55, No. 1 (March), pp. 154–8.

ARROW, K. J. (1968) 'The Economics of Moral Hazard: Further Comment', *American Economic Review*, Vol. 58, No. 3 (June), pp. 537–9.

COOPER, M. H. and CULYER, A. J. (1973) (eds) *Health Economics*. Harmondsworth: Penguin.

CULYER, A. J. (1971) 'Medical Care and the Economics of Giving', *Economica*, Vol. 38, No. 151 (August), pp. 295–303.

DOLBEAR, F. T. (1967) 'On the Theory of Optimal Externality', *American Economic Review*, Vol. 57, No. 1 (March), pp. 90–103.

GREEN, H. A. JOHN (1976) *Consumer Theory*, rev. edn. London and Basingstoke: Macmillan.

HOCHMAN, H. H. and RODGERS, J. D. (1969) 'Pareto–Optimal Redistribution', *American Economic Review*, Vol. 59, No. 3 (September), pp. 542–57.

KESSEL, R. A. (1958) 'Price Discrimination in Medicine', *Journal of Law and Economics*, Vol. 1, No. 2 (October), pp. 20–53.

LEES, D. S. (1961) *Health Through Choice* (Hobart Paper No. 14). London: Institute of Economic Affairs.

LEES, D. S. and RICE, R. G. (1965) 'Uncertainty and the Welfare Economics of Medical Care: Comment', *American Economic Review*, Vol. 55, No. 1 (March), pp. 140–54.

LINDSAY, C. M. (1969) 'Medical Care and Economics of Sharing', *Economica*, Vol. 36, No. 144 (November), pp. 351–62; also reprinted as Reading 3 in Cooper and Culyer (1973).

PAULY, M. V. (1968) 'The Economics of Moral Hazard: Comment', *American Economic Review*, Vol. 58, No. 3 (June), pp. 231–7.

PAULY, M. V. (1971) *Medical Care at Public Expense – A Study in Applied Welfare Economics*. New York: Praeger.

SHIBATA, H. (1971) 'A Bargaining Model of the Pure Theory of Public Expenditure', *Journal of Political Economy*, Vol. 79, No. 1 (January/February), pp. 1–29.

WILLIAMS, A. (1966) 'The Optimal Provision of Public Goods in a System of Local Government', *Journal of Political Economy*, Vol. 74, No. 1 (February), pp. 18–33.

PART II
Health Care Demand Issues

4 The Demand for Health Care

> When an economist talks about the demand for medical care, or any other good or service, he is talking about a willingness and ability to pay. This term should not be confused with 'need' or 'want' or 'desire', although these words are frequently used interchangeably with 'demand' by lay persons. The concept of 'need' for medical care seems to me to be imprecise, and of little value for analytical purposes. In practice it can cover everything from a lifesaving emergency operation to the removal of blackheads.
>
> *V. R. Fuchs* (1968, p. 190)

4.1 Introduction

In Chapter 1 we showed the rapid growth over recent years in the expenditure of resources on health care in Britain, the United States and other countries. This chapter must be viewed against that background, since hand in hand with the greater provision of care is some associated growth in the demand for health care resources. A greater understanding of such demands is essential if any conclusion is to be drawn about the future effects on social welfare of such trends in expenditure. Furthermore, aside from aggregate welfare effects, there may be serious equity problems concerning the allocation of scarce resources in the face of growing demands. Therefore, in this chapter and the next we examine the approaches that have been developed to provide a theory of demand for health care. The implications of each model for social policy and market operation are then considered. Finally, we review the empirical evidence on health care demands.

4.2 Consumer choice and the demand for health care

The foundation on which the whole of demand theory is based is the assumption that the individual consumer is capable of making a rational choice between alternative bundles of goods and services in order to maximise his utility. This choice, as we noted at the start of this book, leads the consumer to demand a quantity of a good or service such that the marginal value of the good equals the price paid. The marginal value of a good in money terms is its marginal utility divided by the marginal utility of money. Thus, utility units are standardised into pounds sterling or dollars, and become the familiar demand curve showing the price a consumer would pay for successive units of the good.

There are several good reasons for arguing that the normal paradigm of a rational utility-maximizing consumer is inappropriate for the health care market. In particular, the consumer's knowledge of his actual state of health and the effects of alternative treatments on that state is likely to diverge from the conventional assumptions of consumer theory. But different implications follow from different assumptions concerning the extent of the divergence between the consumer's conventional theoretical position and the actual situation in the market for health care. The literature of health economics embraces a wide spectrum of demand models. At one extreme the consumer is viewed as having the capacity and information to choose his state of health at all times. At the other, the consumer is seen as lacking any ability to make a choice beyond a yes/no decision dictated by a budget constraint. In order to provide an overview of the range of approaches we consider here the polar cases and one intermediate model.

4.3 The demand for health

The major theoretical innovation in the study of the demand for health care has come from Grossman (1972a, 1972b)[1]. This research goes beyond the obvious but often overlooked point that the demand for health care is *derived* from a demand for health itself (a fundamental commodity in Becker's (1965) terms), to construct a human capital model of consumer behaviour in which the area of choice is extended to choice over state of health.

Grossman's model assumes that individuals assess the benefits from outlays that will improve their health compared with expenditure on other goods and services in order to decide their optimal health state. Consumers are assumed to have knowledge of their own health state, its rate of depreciation and the production function relating health improvements to health care expenditure. Thus, in a world of certainty they choose their lengths of life!

In common with the usual theoretical framework for investment decisions, individuals are assumed to maximise an intertemporal utility function made up of the flow of services from health and consumption of other goods in each year of life. Maximisation leads the individual to equate the marginal return on the asset, health, with its marginal cost. The return to the *j*th individual is made up of the marginal psychic return (a_j) and the marginal monetary return (γ_j). The cost of health capital is the rate of interest forgone on other assets (r_j) plus the rate of depreciation (δ_j) (less any saving from purchase of 'health' now, rather than in the future, owing to future increases in the marginal cost of health improvement). Thus,

$$\gamma_j + a_j = r_j + \delta_j \tag{4.1}$$

for a given consumer in time period *i*.

Grossman examined the consumption and pecuniary investment aspects separately. For simplicity we concentrate here on the investment part of the model only. The pecuniary return (γ_j) depends on three components: the daily wage rate of our representative individual in the *i*th year (W_j^i), the marginal product of health, measured in terms of the number of days of good health generated by a unit of health stock (G_j^i), and the marginal cost of gross investment in health (C_j^{i-1}) purchased in the previous period and including both time and money costs. These three elements combine to give the rate of return:

$$\frac{W_j^i G_j^i}{C_j^{i-1}} = \gamma_j^i = r_j^i + \delta_i^i. \tag{4.2}$$

For any given individual with a given health state there will be an associated marginal product of health *G*. Thus we could plot out a marginal efficiency of health capital schedule showing the return to each level of health $(W_j^i G_j^i)/C_j^{i-1}$. If we assume that the marginal product of health declines asymptoticly to zero as health increases, this curve will have the shape familiar in macroeconomics. Grossman supports such an assumption by pointing out that the return to health, measured in healthy days, has a limit of 365 days per year. This copes with the reduction in disability but not with debility (Chapter 2). The latter may affect wage rates but this problem is explicitly not pursued in the model.

Given the optimal stock of health capital, defined by equation (4.2), we can examine the separate effects of age and income on the optimal stock. Considering age first, assume that wage rates, the marginal product of health stock and the marginal cost of gross investment are independent of age. The assumed effect of increased age is an increase in the rate of depreciation of health (δ_j^i). This is not to suggest that all aged individuals are necessarily less healthy than all young ones, but that for a given individual the annual rate of depreciation of health is greater in old age. The implication of Grossman's assumptions is that, from equation (4.2), increased depreciation leads the consumer to choose a lower stock of health in order to increase the marginal product of health and equate the marginal return with the higher cost. (We have already assumed that the marginal product of health is lower the higher the health stock.) Thus, when faced with known and increasing rates of health depreciation, Grossman's model suggests that the individual will *choose* a lower health state in each successive year. This leads him to choose his length of life as the optimal health stock will ultimately decline below some necessary life-supporting minimum and death will occur.

The demand for health care is derived from the demand for an optimal health stock in each period, with current health stock, depreciation and investment in health care being the determinants of future health stock. But the health stock and the flow of gross investment are not simply related. Declining health stock over time is not necessarily associated with declining consumption of health care in each year. The increasing depreciation rate reduces the net increase in health from a unit of gross investment through health care. That is, the additional health created is subject to the same higher depreciation rate as the existing stock and so less net investment is produced per unit of gross investment. The precise relationship between age and health care consumption depends on the elasticity of the demand for health. This will be highly inelastic if the marginal product of health rises rapidly as health state falls; e.g., if a small reduction in a particular individual's health state owing to depreciation prevents him working at all when previously he worked full-time, then the marginal product of a small increase in health will be very large. Thus, in the face of a higher cost of health owing to increased depreciation, he will purchase additional health care to offset the depreciation. His new health state will thus be close to his original state (see Figure 4.1(a)). Conversely, if a reduction in health has a smaller effect on the marginal product of health, then the individual will not seek to offset a great deal of the natural depreciation in his state of health. Therefore, when his health state falls he may seek less health care (see Figure 4.1(b)).

The two diagrams together make this point more simply. Both individuals start at point 1. Over a year their health state depreciates by the same proportion and the rate of depreciation increases to put them at point 2. Both respond according to their demand curves – the marginal efficiency of health capital – to the new higher marginal cost of health. In Figure 4.1(a) a large part of the depreciation is offset by health care while in (b) it is not. Both arrive at point 3. In subsequent periods, as depreciation rates increase, an individual behaving as in Figure 4.1(a) suffers bigger losses of health stock, as his absolute level is higher, and

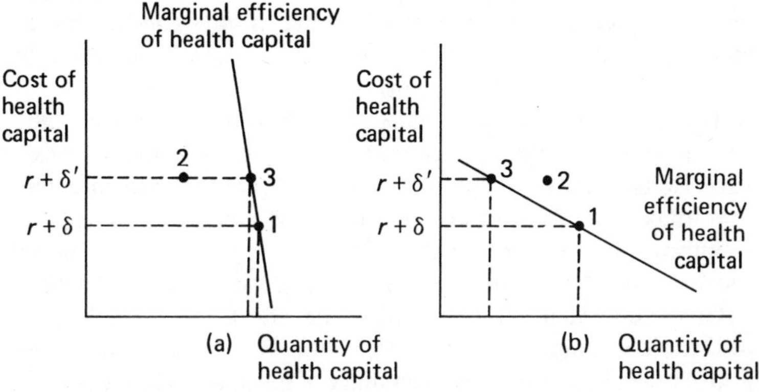

Figure 4.1 Health stock responses to increased depreciation

invests more in health care to offset the fall, as the amount of health produced per unit of health care falls with rising depreciation. It should be clear that the opposite outcome occurs if the individual's demand for health is elastic as in Figure 4.1(b).

The effect of wage rates on the stock of health and the demand for care is made up from two elements. The marginal product of health, measured in healthy days, is clearly worth more at higher wage rates. But the consumer's time is also an input into health care, and so, if the wage rate increases by Z per cent, then the cost of care will increase by

$$\frac{Wt}{Wt + P_h} \cdot Z < Z$$

where W = wage rate
t = time input per unit health care
P_h = price per unit of other inputs to health care.

Assuming that own time is not the only health care input, the percentage increase in wages will exceed the increase in unit cost and the return to health will increase at all levels of health stock. That is, the marginal efficiency schedule or demand for health will shift upwards, causing higher levels of health to be demanded at any given interest and depreciation rates. The precise impact of higher wages depends on the elasticity of the demand for health and the share of time costs in total unit cost of health care. However, since the increment of health obtained from a unit of gross investment in health care is not affected by the increase in wages, the demand for health care will increase (or, in the extreme, remain constant) with rising wage rates.

The health capital model has few implications for public policy to improve the efficiency or equity of the provision of health care. Consumers are taken to be capable of making efficient choices that maximise their utility. Health care consumption is likely to increase with income, and so, since consumer choice is efficient, income support measures will achieve the desired degree of equity.[2]

Grossman went on to examine the effects of education and also the consumption benefits of health. But the brief discussion above provides a convenient summary of his approach. Its explanatory success is an empirical matter, to which we return later when comparing its predictions with other, simpler models, but it is noteworthy that it offers no surprising predictions in spite of its complexity. However, before leaving Grossman it is worth emphasising, as Dowie (1975) has, that perhaps the major public policy role to be filled by government in a Grossman-type world is the provision of health information on the effects of detrimental health inputs and on efficiency in combining favourable inputs rather than the provision of health services *per se*. This follows from the individual, and not doctors, hospitals and the like, being the 'producer' of the commodity health.

4.4 The demand for health care

The implications of a relatively simple theoretical framework form the focus of this section. It concerns the sensitivity of consumer demand to the various components of the cost of obtaining health care. We have already noted the fact that health care consumption typically requires significant inputs of the consumer's time. A further aspect is that the cost of care is frequently covered by insurance. (A 'free' public health system effectively insures the individual against all costs but charges a tax 'premium' to finance them.) Therefore, aside from direct responses to price changes we are also interested in the possible effects of various insurance schemes on the aggregate demand for health care.

Phelps and Newhouse (1974) modelled the behaviour of a utility-maximising individual whose expenditure on health care is covered by a very simple form of insurance. After paying an initial fixed premium the consumer is covered for a fixed percentage of the cost of health care regardless of the quantity consumed – a co-payment scheme. Thus, the consumer pays CP_h per unit of health care, where P_h is the market price and C the proportion of the cost of care for which the consumer is liable. In addition, each unit of health care consumed requires an input of the consumer's time t which is valued at an opportunity cost W per unit time. The total cost of health care is therefore $(CP_h + Wt)$ per unit.

The health state of the individual is assumed to be random, hence his willingness to insure against the costs. Once insured, (i.e. after the fixed insurance payment has been made for the time period in question) the individual maximises his utility from treatment when ill by choosing the quantity of health care that equalises the marginal value of care and its marginal cost, $(CP_h + Wt)$. Let this quantity be h. The quantity chosen by the consumer is assumed to respond to changes in the total cost of care $(CP_h + Wt)$ with some elasticity, η. Without inquiring directly into this, Phelps and Newhouse treated it as a constant and examined the elasticity of demand with respect to the components of total cost per unit. That is, they considered the four elasticities of demand with respect to price (η_{hP_h}), share of costs borne by the consumer, (η_{hC}), time input per unit of health care (η_{ht}) and opportunity cost of time (η_{hW}).

It can be shown[3] that the model leads to the following elasticities:

$$\eta_{hP_h} \doteq \eta_{hC} \doteq \frac{CP_h}{CP_h + Wt}\eta \tag{4.3}$$

$$\eta_{ht} \doteq \eta_{hW} \doteq \frac{Wt}{CP_h + Wt}\eta \tag{4.4}$$

That is, the elasticity of demand with respect to the components of the money cost of treatment is approximately equal to the elasticity of demand with respect to the total cost of care per unit multiplied by the proportion of the total cost per unit made up by money cost. Similarly, for time cost the elasticity with respect to total cost per unit is multiplied by the proportion made up by time costs. Thus, if we accept the elasticity η as a fixed datum of consumer behaviour, we can derive implications based on the components of total cost per unit. These cover not only the effects of variations in insurance arrangements but also the differential effects of changes in the components of total cost per unit in different fields of medicine. Health care treatment varies in the amount of own time required from taking an aspirin to major surgery, and so the sensitivity of demand for care of different kinds to changes in the time cost will vary.

We wish to concentrate there on the implications as they relate to the known expansion of expenditure on health care. Demand for treatments that are not time-intensive but money–price-intensive (i.e. $[(CP_h)/(CP_h + Wt)] > [(Wt)/(CP_h + Wt)]$) are likely to be more sensitive to the introduction of insurance cover or free provision. Conversely, the demand for time-intensive treatment will be more responsive to technical changes in required time inputs or economic changes in the opportunity cost of time. The former type of health care is the sort provided by home visits by general practitioners where the patient sacrifices little or no useful time while being prescribed and taking the treatment. By implication, the latter type of care is provided by hospital in-patient services which require prolonged periods of inactivity. But Phelps and Newhouse have noted a further difficulty here. In-patient treatment is typically required for the more serious diseases, and when suffering from these the patient is already restricted in his activity. Thus, the opportunity cost of time in these cases may not be particularly high and the demand response to changes in time cost unimportant. Perhaps the most likely form of treatment to have a high time cost share of total unit cost is treatment that can be provided by the individual for himself or by health care services. The time saved by self-care would outweigh the money saved by receiving care from an insurance or state funded supplier, e.g. for treating minor cuts and bruises. Some limited empirical evidence exists for the UK and will be discussed below.

The predictions of the model are in general that money price reductions in the cost of care are important influences on the quantity of care demanded, time price effects being relevant for a smaller set of disorders and forms of care. The implications of this model for policy are that a reduction in the cost of health care at the time of purchase will increase demand beyond the level that would be efficient in a pure market. Thus, efficiency would require the restriction of demand by the institutions of the supply side of the market. But we will discuss later the lack of incentive to take such action in a private market. A public policy in which rationing is applied to the supply of care is an alternative to which we return. On equity grounds, income support would again remedy any inequality regarded as socially undesirable. The alternative strategy of publicly funded care would increase demand and might require rationing to prevent inefficiency owing to the expansion in demand.

Although the Phelps and Newhouse model approaches the reality of the consumer's decision more closely than the health stock models, many critics of health economics would still regard it as unsatisfactory. In the model health care is assessed and consumed by the individual in a way similar to consumer choice over goods where the consumer is well equipped for choice by prior knowledge of the product or experience of consuming it. But critics typically argue that the individual has a 'need' for treatment rather than a desire or demand for it. Therefore, we turn to a framework that reduces further the emphasis placed on the consumer's freedom of choice.

4.5 Need versus demand

Assume initially that the typical consumer of health care has no information or ability with which to forecast his state of health other than the obvious expectation that his health will generally decline with age. Each period of ill health, which we define as any pain or restriction of activity which the individual regards as abnormal for his age, cultural norms, sex, social class etc., takes the individual by surprise. He seeks medical advice in order to find out what further action he should take. But since we have assumed that he has no knowledge of the links between treatment and the characteristics he desires, the restoration of his activities and relief from pain (see p. 40), the treatment decision lies exclusively with the doctor. It is the doctor who decides the quantity and type of health care appropriate and also, in general, supplies some or all of the care. The only decision left to the consumer is a take-it-or-leave-it one. He has to decide how much the relief of pain and restoration of activity are worth to him. Note that this is their total value and not their marginal value. The treatment is offered as a single package and the patient is assumed to accept the doctor's judgement that the whole package is the appropriate one. (Half an operation or half a course of antibiotics is useless.) If the total value of the benefits of treatment exceeds the cost of the package, then the consumer will purchase the health care recommended. Alternatively, if the value placed on the benefits is less than the total cost then he will decline treatment.

This approach is termed the 'needs' approach because the consumer does not demand care on his own initiative. His need for care is assessed by his doctor in terms of the quantity of care that will restore, as far as possible, the individual's health to the level the doctor expects. That is, need for health care is defined as the medical assessment of the treatment necessary to bring the patient to a medically assessed standard of health. (For an elegant and comprehensive review of the various meanings of 'need', see Williams, 1974). The amount of care recommended to the patient will thus depend on the diagnosis of his condition, the medical technology available to treat it and the doctor's choice of technique.

The implication of the discussion so far is that, when suffering from a particular illness, the individual has an effective demand curve for care that is totally inelastic (see Figure 4.2). He 'chooses' *Oh* units of health care because this is his doctor's choice, and he will pay up to the amount shown by area $OP_h'\beta h$ for them, this being the total value he places on the benefit predicted by his doctor. Therefore, if the cost of care, price OP_h times quantity *Oh* (i.e. $OP_h\alpha h$) is less than $OP_h'\beta h$ then he purchases the prescribed course of treatment.

The inelasticity of the demand for health care is implicit in

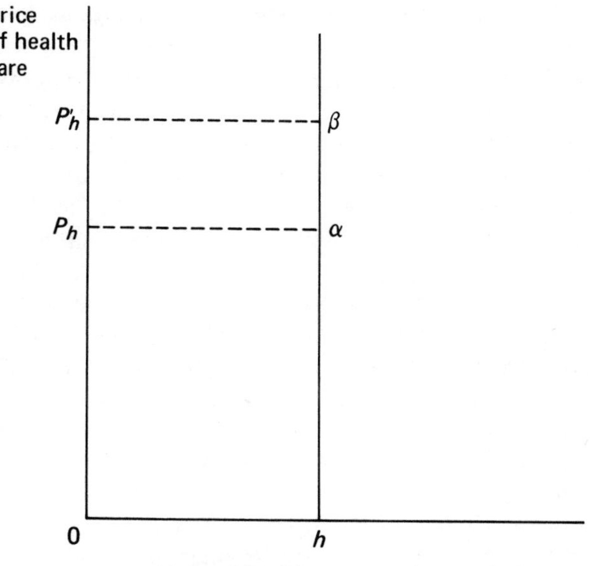

Figure 4.2 Need as inelastic demand

the argument for providing a free and universal national health service in order to protect those who cannot 'afford' the appropriate care for their disease. These are individuals whose total valuation of treatment is limited by a budget constraint to a figure lower than the cost of treatment. We have already examined some methods of helping the poor. At this stage, however, we depart from the earlier analysis of alternative methods of dealing with supplementation for the poor. Instead we focus on the need-based inelastic demand curve.

The inelasticity of demand essentially removes the standard textbook argument against the unrestricted free provision of a good for individual consumption. This is the efficiency argument that free provision to all, although equitable, will encourage consumption up to the level at which the marginal utility of the good to the consumer is zero. Although society may (but may not) wish to expand consumption by the poor to this level, it is inefficient if any individual's consumption at the margin yields benefits to himself and the rest of society totalling less than the marginal cost of provision. Figure 4.3 indicates such inefficiency for one rich (A) and one poor (B) consumer when demand is elastic. Left to their own devices they would consume Oh_A and Oh_B units of health care. If individual B is subsidised in some way to take account of the benefits to others of an improvement in his health, his demand curve shifts to D_B' and he chooses Oh_B' units of health care. If to avoid the difficulties of personal subsidies and means tests health care is supplied free of charge and without rationing, both increase their consumption, to Oh_B'' and Oh_A'. Individual A's consumption is inefficiently large in that he consumes some health care that he values at less than the marginal cost to society of supplying it. B's consumption is also inefficiently high even when society's view of his consumption is included since it exceeds Oh_B'. It is possible that his consumption at zero price will equal the socially optimal quantity if his demand curve has the correct shape but this will occur only by chance. It is much more likely that his demand will be inefficiently high, since at zero price the monetary reasons for his demand being less than the rich man's are removed. Therefore, income supplements are preferred on efficiency grounds to free unrestricted provision. Chapter 3 has already examined such issues for health care, but on the assumption of an elastic demand curve. If the

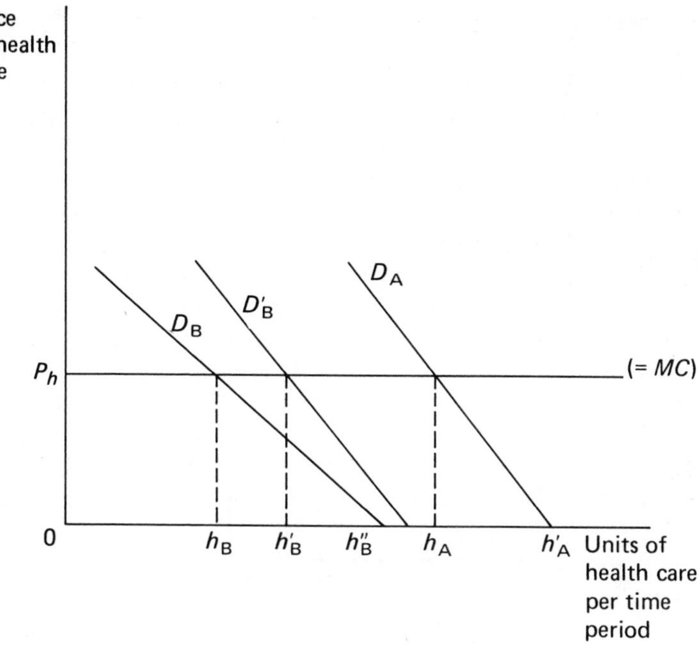

Figure 4.3 Demand responses to zero prices

needs model is correct, there is no quantity response to the lowering of price and so the inefficiency is eliminated. Those who previously could not afford the prescribed treatment now receive the same quantity free of charge. Equity will thus be achieved, if the health care provided is financed by an equitable tax structure, while the efficiency of resource allocation to health care provision is not impaired.

However, the needs argument cannot be regarded as providing an unambiguous policy recommendation that free health care is an efficient method of meeting the health needs of the poor, because so far we have *failed* to establish that demand is inelastic. What we have demonstrated is that the consumer, when suffering from a given disease, has an inelastic demand for treatment for that disease because he accepts that the course of treatment recommended by his doctor is the correct one. But what if our individual over a year suffers from a whole range of disorders causing some pain and/or some disability? We can rank the diseases according to the valuation he places on the relief of each one. In Figure

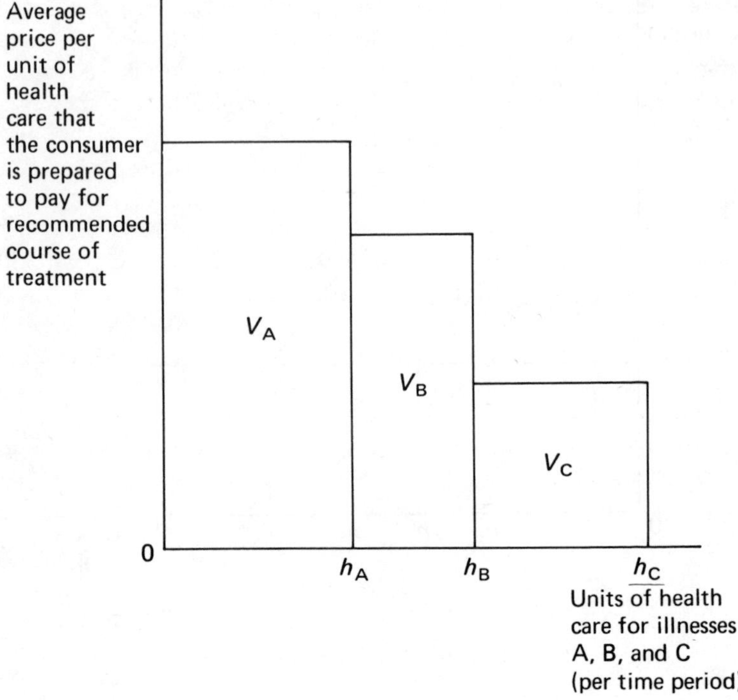

Figure 4.4 Need and demand with more than one disease per time period

4.4 areas (V_A), (V_B), (V_C) etc. show the maximum amount the patient will pay for Oh_A, $h_A h_B$ and $h_B h_C$ units of health care where these are the quantities of treatment prescribed for diseases A, B, C. By the introduction of more than one disease affecting the individual in the relevant period we have produced a demand for health care that is elastic, the quantity demanded increasing as the price falls. Such a demand curve would lead both rich and poor to consume a quantity of health care at zero price that was inefficient; i.e., the total value to the consumer and the rest of society of some courses of treatment would be less than their total cost. Therefore our initial needs model, where the consumer has no choice other than a yes/no decision on purchasing the complete course of treatment, does not ensure that demand is totally inelastic. Nor does it lead us to reject the conventional demand framework for health care or the arguments on the inefficiency of 'free' provision. Instead, it effectively reinstates demand because of the quantity response to a lower price. This leads to inefficiencies in the consumption of 'free' public care, because provision at zero price does not merely permit the poor to increase their consumption of health care that previously cost more than their total health care budget; it also encourages both rich and poor to demand treatment that was previously not demanded because its value to the consumer was less than the private market cost. Thus, many treatments that are curing medically trivial complaints at relatively high cost will be demanded when 'free' provision exists. The implication is that for efficiency reasons the demand for health care must be restricted, by price or other means, because the demand for care is not totally inelastic.

To summarise, the policy implications of the discussion so far in this chapter are that 'free' unrestricted provision will be equitable but inefficient, and that market provision coupled with specific support for the poor, e.g. as discussed in Chapter 3, will be a more advantageous policy. But the efficiency of the market is no longer clear-cut when consumers cannot rationally assess the quantity they require. Therefore, we consider next the effects of supplier behaviour on demand. This discussion is not deferred until the chapters on supply because it is central to an understanding of the growth of demand. However, in our discussion of supply later, we have to introduce some further dimensions of demand, since the absence of consumer knowledge of the product links supplier and consumer inextricably.

4.6 Supplier-induced demand

The needs model proposed that consumers would purchase the amount of health care prescribed by their doctor as long as its total cost fell within some total cost constraint. If the consumer does not shop around then the supplier of health care can increase the price or quantity of care provided to the consumer arbitrarily as long as he does not exceed this constraint. This leads us to question the determinants of the all-important budget constraint. For a 'selfish' utility-maximiser, i.e. a consumer whose utility is wholly unaffected by the welfare of others, the income constraint in the case of emergency potential life-saving care is likely to approach his total wealth and, in the unlikely event of loans being available to finance such treatment, to exceed it. Only if a life of abject poverty or the lower wealth of dependents (i.e. all those whose future welfare enters the consumer's utility function) is deemed worse than death will the budget constraint be a sum less than total wealth. For less serious disorders the consumer will assess the value of the predicted benefits of treatment. The greater the certainty with which they are forecast and the greater the relief of symptoms and restoration of normal activity, the higher the budget constraint is likely to be.

Income is also likely to have a positive effect on the health care cost constraint for a number of reasons. The rich can offer a higher total wealth for emergency, potential life-saving care. They can also offer to purchase more of all goods and services. Finally, higher income also increases the individual's range of recreation activities, which in turn increases the opportunity cost of restrictions owing to illness.

Education, aside from its effects on income, is likely to increase the budget constraint in so far as the individual learns the importance of early diagnosis of chronic conditions, for example. In addition, the consumer's acquisition of knowledge about his disorder may have a profound effect on the amount he is prepared to pay since it alters his perception of the benefits of treatment. Of course, it is impossible to assert that these factors will be important for all consumers. Indeed, the major weakness of the economist's theory of consumer behaviour is that it formalises choice behaviour without predicting it to any great extent. (E.g., a price cut may cause a consumer to buy more of a commodity – substitution effect – or less – income effect).

The supplier of health care in a market regime can increase the demand for health care by gaining information on the factors that influence the consumer's willingness to pay for relief from a particular disorder. While he is unlikely to have direct access to data on patient incomes, data on residential location, education and occupation are likely to be readily provided by the patient. This enables the supplier to estimate willingness to pay by proxy, since such data correlate strongly with income. The discouragement of overt competition, price cutting and advertising, and restrictions on the output of medical schools, are further methods for ensuring that patients always pay an amount as close to the maximum as can be achieved. The quality of care sought by suppliers and consumers is a further influence, which we discuss in detail in Chapter 6 on supply.

An environment of rising real income, coupled with consumers who do not directly demand care but behave according to the need framework, provides an opportunity for supplier-induced demand to increase. The consumers' response is to seek insurance which will provide care at a cost less than the maximum he is prepared to pay. But insurance cover also removes the risk of the supplier exceeding the patient's budget constraint when recommending a course of treatment, since the patient is more likely to reveal the extent of his insurance cover, not least as a guarantee of payment for high-cost treatment. Insurance companies then become the central controllers of expenditure, determining their own cover in relation to fixed price schedules and the price elasticity of their income from insurance premiums. But here again, it is only when premiums approach the consumer's willingness to spend on health care when suffering from disease in the future time period that any resistance to rising expenditure develops. Thus, the relationship between supplier income and supplier-prescribed demand will tend to produce a situation in which a high degree of price discrimination operates and in which willingness to pay, regardless of the actual incidence of disease, generates additional expenditure on health care.

Of course, it would be disingenuous to suggest that the removal of the key link between suppliers' incomes and their prescription of treatment would secure an unambiguous improvement for the consumer. Too little treatment, rather than too much, may result. But certainly it is clear that, if consumers are indeed in the position outlined immediately above, conventional demand theory and its implications for intervention in the market cannot be accepted.

Supplier-induced demand certainly provides a theoretical case for market intervention in the same way as monopoly. Consumers pay more for treatment than is necessary because of the doctor's monopoly of knowledge and the indivisibility of courses of treatment. They forgo the consumption of additional goods and services, this being transferred to their doctors as a monopoly rent over and above the amount necessary to keep them in the market.

To prevent consumer exploitation it would be necessary to devise some mechanism for removing the incentive to over-provide treatment or charge higher prices. A public health care system in which supply is rationed to the level of care consistent with efficiency is one solution. An alternative is price-fixing in the health care market by government or insurance companies, together with supervision of the quantity of care provided. Further discussion of both these policies will be found in Chapters 10 and 11.

4.7 Summary

This chapter has covered a wide range of demand theories in order to demonstrate the implications for policy. These can be summarised by the statement that 'the greater the consumer's ability to choose, the less the importance of intervention to achieve efficiency'. At one extreme the consumer is viewed as capable of planning his health state, subject to some random fluctuations from the planned pattern, because he has knowledge of the effects of health care on his health state and the rate at which his health deteriorates. (In this model man was seen basically as a depreciating capital good capable of improvement by net investment.) Even when the consumer has less choice, choosing the quantity of care when he is ill, the case for intervention is weak. Equity considerations can be resolved by income support for the poor when the ability to choose exists. But in other circumstances it is essential that further controls on the operation of the market be introduced, particularly if the supplier is the prime mover in the market place. In examining the empirical evidence that follows, the reader should bear in mind that all the approaches in this chapter are consistent with similar evidence. Income and education are both likely to be positively correlated with expenditure on medical care, since, regardless of the consumer's knowledge and ability to choose, both can be expected to contribute directly or indirectly to expanding budget constraints. In addition, education is likely to increase the awareness of the consumer of health and health care. Therefore, the evidence that follows cannot be taken as direct confirmation of any particular model. However, we will argue that, taken with a realistic appraisal of the theories of demand, supplier-induced demand is the most sensible framework for policy. The 'needs' model was discussed in terms of need as inelastic demand indicated by the physician; however, for policy discussions in the social policy fields, alternative concepts of need have to be developed, an example of which is briefly described in the Appendix to this chapter.

Appendix: 'Need' and social policy discussions

In the social policy field in general and the health care field in particular, people are often said to be in 'need'. It is not often clear what is meant by this term; hence some relatively recent studies have attempted to give precise content to the term 'need'. As noted above, a summary can be found in Williams (1974); nevertheless a brief example is provided here as indicative of these studies.

Spek (1972) and Bradshaw (1972) have both developed 'need' frameworks that revolve around establishing precisely who is saying (or doing) what about (to) whom. Spek's (1972) formulation involves three parties: society, medical experts and the individual himself, answering the questions 'is the individual sick?' and 'Is the individual in need of public care?' A third question, 'Does the individual demand public care?', enables Spek to complete his taxonomy. Bradshaw suggests that in practice four separate definitions of need are used by social policy researchers and practitioners (examples here are provided with reference to health care but they could come from any social service).

(a) *Normative need* occurs where people have a standard of health care below that which the health care expert defines as desirable. It must be noted that this 'desirable' standard may vary between experts.

(b) *Felt need* occurs where people want health care; i.e., it relates to the individual's perceptions as regards health care, which clearly may conflict with others' views of their wants, e.g. hypochondriacs.

(c) *Expressed need* is felt need converted into demand, for example by seeking health care from a National Health Service doctor (demand here is not necessarily the economist's notion, which involves a willingness and ability to pay for a service).

(d) *Comparative need* occurs where one group in society with given health characteristics does not receive health care whereas others with identical characteristics are in receipt of care.

These four definitions are interrelated and can be used to give twelve possible combinations of need configurations. If +1 indicates the presence of need on definition 1 and −1 the absence of need on definition 1, etc., then −1, +2, +3 and +4 would mean the individual is in receipt of health care not thought to be necessary by the expert but that is wanted, demanded by the individual and received by others in similar circumstances; for example some forms of cosmetic surgery. +1, −2, −3, +4 could represent the situation where there is a clinical iceberg of ill health, i.e. where expert opinion thinks care is appropriate and some in society with a given set of characteristics receive care; however many in society with identical characteristics do not want or demand care. Population surveys often reveal large numbers of people who have identifiable illnesses but do not want (perceive they need) or demand health care; e.g., Last (1963) estimated that for epilepsy there were six unrecognised cases in the average general practice of 2250 people in England and Wales in 1960. Although it is easy to see how such a need taxonomy may facilitate research and policy analysis, the policy-maker is still left with the unenviable task of deciding what part of the total need described under the various headings is 'real' need and therefore worth attempting to alleviate.

Until recently it was the practice for economists to avoid the word 'need' in their language and analysis. Now, however, some at least take the concept seriously and are concerned with deriving definitions of need and exploring the roles of values in health status measurement. For example, Culyer (1978) has defined need as either (a) the potential for *avoidance* of reductions in health status or (b) the potential for *improvements* in health status above the level it would otherwise reach. Culyer has also explored the role of value judgements in the choice of dimensions in which to measure health status, the choice of weights to be used in trading off different dimensions of health status against each other and the final choice of a cardinal number to be assigned to each combination of health status dimensions. For a summary of the root of much of this literature, see Section 8.7.

NOTES

1. Grossman (1972b) excludes empirical results.
2. Equity is discussed in more detail in Chapter 11; however, we have in mind a situation in which the receipt of health care is determined by (ill) health status rather than income, social class and the like.
3. See Phelps and Newhouse (1973).

REFERENCES

BECKER, G. S. (1965) 'A Theory of the Allocation of Time', *Economic Journal*, Vol. 75, No. 299 (September), pp. 493–517.

BRADSHAW, J. (1972) 'A Taxonomy of Social Need', pp. 69–82 in McLachlan, G. (ed.) *Problems and Progress in Medical Care* (Essays in Current Research, 7th Series). London: Oxford University Press for the National Provincial Hospitals Trust.

CULYER, A. J. (1978) 'Need, Values and Health Status Measurement', Chapter 2, pp. 9–31, in Culyer, A. J. and Wright, K. G. (eds), *Economic Aspects of Health Services*. London: Martin Robertson.

DOWIE, J. (1975) 'The Portfolio Approach to Health Behaviour', *Social Science and Medicine*, Vol. 9, No. 11/12 (November/December), pp. 619–31.

FUCHS, V. R. (1968) 'The Growing Demand for Medical Care', *New England Journal of Medicine*, Vol. 279, No. 192 (25 July), pp. 190–5; reprinted as Chapter 4, pp. 61–8 in Fuchs, V. R. (ed.), (1972) *Essays in the Economics of Health and Medical Care*, New York and London: Columbia University Press for National Bureau of Economic Research.

GROSSMAN, M. (1972a) *The Demand for Health: a Theoretical and Empirical Investigation* (National Bureau of Economic Research Occasional Paper 119). New York and London: Columbia University Press.

GROSSMAN, M. (1972b) 'On the Concept of Health Capital and the Demand for Health', *Journal of Political Economy*, Vol. 80, No. 2 (March/April), pp. 223–55.

LAST, J. M. (1963) '"The Iceberg": Completing the Clinical Picture in General Practice', *Lancet*, Vol. 2, No. 7297 (6 July), pp. 28–31.

PHELPS, C. E. and NEWHOUSE, J. P. (1973) *Coinsurance and the Demand for Medical Services*. Santa Monica, California: Rand Corporation.

PHELPS, C. E. and NEWHOUSE, J. P. (1974) 'Coinsurance, the Price of Time and the Demand for Medical Services', *Review of Economics and Statistics*, Vol. 56, No. 3 (August), pp. 334–42.

SPEK, J. E. (1972) 'On the Economic Analysis of Health and Medical Care in a Swedish Health District', pp. 261–8 in Hauser, M. M. (ed.) *The Economics of Medical Care*, London: George Allen & Unwin.

WILLIAMS, A. (1974) '"Need" as a Demand Concept (with special reference to health)', Chapter 4, pp. 60–78 in Culyer, A. J. (ed.) *Economic Policies and Social Goals: Aspects of Public Choice*, London: Martin Robertson.

5 Empirical Evidence on the Demand for Health Care

> . . . it is my hope that more economists in this country will respond to the challenge of devising 'demand' functions which will isolate the relative extents to which money, time, knowledge, energy and desperation (health status? tastes? needs? ability to pay?) influence the health-care-seeking behaviour of different groups in the community.
>
> *A. Williams* (1977, pp. 309–10)

5.1 Introduction

In this chapter we examine the empirical evidence produced by the authors of models that broadly conform to one of the approaches reviewed in the previous chapter. The empirical formulations of the models are frequently confronted by difficulties of measurement requiring considerable ingenuity to overcome them. However, since our interest here is in the results rather than in the techniques used to obtain them, we present only a brief discussion of methodology, concentrating instead on the characteristics of each study and its outcome.

Throughout we focus also on the policy relevance of the results. In particular this concerns the extent to which the rapid increases in expenditure on health care can be explained by conventional demand or by other factors such as insurance or supplier behaviour.[1] While growth of demand because of consumer tastes is unlikely to concern policy-makers, inefficiencies owing to demand expansion for other reasons are clearly of interest to politicians seeking equity and efficiency in health care provision.

Finally, the reader should note that almost all the evidence in this chapter comes from studies of North America. In the UK almost all health care has been free of direct money cost since 1948, and so conventional economic explanations are of only limited interest. Rather we need to look at the behaviour of the dominant group, the suppliers, which in our view is of fundamental importance to an understanding of increasing health expenditure not only in the UK but also in the USA. (The problem is a much larger one in the USA: see Chapter 11 for statistical evidence on its extent.)

5.2 Problems of demand estimation

A rapid increase in expenditure on a particular good can be explained within the framework of simple demand theory by a number of causal factors. The simplest of these is the price of the good. A rise in price increases expenditure when the demand is inelastic while a fall in price produces the same effect when demand is elastic. Thus, when examining expenditure on health care in a market system of supply, the price of care is of major interest. However, the difficulty in assessing price effects in the field of health care is that health care is a highly heterogeneous product with a range of different prices. Where expenditure data rather than quantity data are available no simple standardisation by a price index is possible without some mis-estimation of the exact quantities involved. A number of studies have been able to circumvent this difficulty by obtaining data on the precise use of homogeneous units of care such as days of stay in hospital. But expenditure data are more widely available for consumers who may be unaware of the precise details of care received. Income received by suppliers of different sorts may be more useful, but again only if a price deflator is available.

A further difficulty is that observations on price and quantity of a good purchased in successive time periods or across different locations do not of themselves map out a demand curve. Each observation shows the intersection of a demand and a supply for one place at one point of time. Observations for different points in time or different locations will depend on temporary and local demand curves which are unlikely to be identical to the original. Therefore, instead of estimating a simple demand curve of the familiar form:

$$Q_D = f(P) \tag{5.1}$$

where Q_D is the quantity demanded and P is the market price, it is necessary to take account of the other variables that will contribute to shifting the demand curve. Our earlier theoretical discussion suggests income (Y), insurance cover (INS), education (ED), age (AGE) and health stock (H) as the important influences on demand. Therefore, the estimated demand equation is typically derived from regression analysis of equations of the form:

$$Q_D = f(P, Y, INS, ED, AGE, H, \ldots). \tag{5.2}$$

Depending on data availability, other variables are included in particular studies e.g. racial origin, family size.

The functional form used in the regression equation varies in each study but is typically linear or log-linear (i.e. regressing the logarithm of expenditure on the log of some or all the independent variables). Other variations include attempts to take account of possible non-linearities in relationships, e.g. by the introduction of the squared value of an independent variable together with the variable itself. (See Chapter 7 for a discussion of this point in the estimation of hospital costs.) The estimated equation provides coefficients on each variable which then enable us to assess the elasticity of demand with respect to it.[2]

Aside from the problems of estimating a consistent demand curve, a further specific difficulty applies to one aspect of the Grossman (1972) model, the demand for health capital. Health state is not directly measurable from survey data or observed market transactions except by individual statements of self-assessed health, which may not be particularly reliable. As an alternative, Grossman uses the amount of healthy time (i.e. 365 days less days of sickness absence) which is a product of the health stock. This permits him to infer the state of health of individuals in the sample and then to regress this on the various independent variables.

5.3 The empirical results

In this section we examine the empirical results of a number of authors concerning each of the relevant variables in turn. The discussion is oriented towards the growth of demand in the recent past and so we examine first the effects of income on demand, since rising real income is a known influence on consumer expenditure. We then examine the effects of (time) price changes, particularly in connection with alternative forms of insurance cover. The limited results on the effects of education are briefly presented. Finally we consider evidence on supplier-induced demand.

5.3.1 Income effects

Estimates provided by Grossman (1972), Rosett and Huang (1973) and Phelps and Newhouse (1974a) all indicate a positive effect of income on health care expenditure. Grossman's results also indicate a negative relationship between income and the individual's number of healthy days per year. This runs counter to the implications of his model and we return to it below.

Grossman and Phelps/Newhouse introduce some measure of the wage rate or wage component of income in addition to the income measure. This takes account of the influence of the wage rate on the time cost of certain types of health care. Both studies confirm that the demand for health care in general, or for certain time-intensive types of care, varies inversely with the wage rate.

The results of the three studies are not strictly comparable because of the different data and different techniques used. Hence, they can be viewed only as a general indication of the responsiveness of demand. All three studies under discussion here, together with a number of earlier ones, suggest that the income elasticity of demand for health care is less than unity, i.e. that a k per cent rise in income leads to an increase in demand of less than k per cent.

At the same time, *this* evidence suggests that income increases alone do not account for the rate of increase of health care consumption in the United States at a pace exceeding the growth rate of incomes. Grossman's results indicate an elasticity of about 0.7 when the negative effect of wage rates is separately accounted for. Phelps and Newhouse report elasticities of 0.1 or less for non-wage income when wage income is included separately in the estimating equation. Rosett and Huang obtained estimates of between 0.25 and 0.45 using no wage adjustments. These results together imply a negative effect of wage rates, giving lower income elasticities when wage rate is not included. This is broadly in line with earlier theoretical discussion.

The negative effect of income on days of good health enjoyed per year found by Grossman leads him to conclude that the effects of luxury good consumption by the rich are damaging to their health, outweighing the beneficial inputs to health production and leading to a lower health stock than would be expected on income grounds alone. The rich effectively trade off their health against the fruits of the good life, alcohol being the most obvious, but by no means the only, such fruit.

It may also be that, in order to achieve a high income, a less 'healthy' job, involving more stress, greater risk of accident and less exercise, must be accepted. This was noted by Auster, Leveson and Sarachek (1969) in their study of the impact of health care and environmental factors (income, education, *per capita* alcohol and cigarette consumption, etc.) on mortality.

In general, although we can put only limited confidence in the precise numerical estimates of income elasticity of demand, the results in the health economics literature suggest that we must examine other causal factors.

The observant reader will be wondering how these results can be reconciled with the estimates of the income elasticity of medical care expenditures reported in Chapter 1. Newhouse (1977) realised that his cross-national results showing health care expenditure to be highly income-elastic ran counter to the evidence of cross-section data within the United States showing low (or negative) income elasticities with respect to medical care expenditure. The explanation of this, according to Newhouse, is that for a given country and point in time money price is often not an important rationing factor (either because of the absence of user charges, e.g. the NHS, or because of extensive insurance cover, e.g. the USA) which in a model developed by Phelps and Newhouse (1974b) implies that the income elasticity will fall.[3] Furthermore, if there is subsidised health care for the poor or price discrimination, the low income elasticity within a country includes a price effect. However, with inter-country comparisons and time series study of a single country the full price of health care has to be faced and income considerations become important.

Having noted how insurance cover reduces the effective price of health care in the United States and how in Britain's NHS money costs are effectively zero, a rational question to which we now turn is the estimated impact this has had on health expenditures and whether it is consistent with the finding that overall income is the main determinant of a nation's health care expenditures. More specifically, the next section examines the price elasticity of demand when insurance cover is introduced.

5.3.2 *Insurance effects*

One difficulty in attempting to assess the impact of insurance cover on the expenditure on an individual's health care is that in the United States the variety of insurance schemes is such that no simple co-insurance rate is readily measurable as a summary of an individual's insurance cover. Rosett and Huang (1973) attempted to infer the effective co-insurance rate, i.e. the amount of the unit cost of health care borne by the insurance company, from the various insurance data on the extent and rate of cover. Their results suggested, as expected, that the co-insurance rate is positively related to the gross expenditure on health care by the consumer (i.e. including expenditure refunded by insurance companies). In addition the results suggested a greater income elasticity of demand the higher the co-insurance rate. This is intuitively highly plausible since the individual with greater insurance cover faces a lower net price of health cover and can afford the cost of a larger amount of health care per dollar increase in income than could an individual with little or no cover.

Phelps and Newhouse (1974a) have reviewed a variety of evidence on insurance effects in connection with their work on time costs and money costs of care. The after-effects of a 25 per cent co-insurance rate introduced in Palo Alto in 1967 indicated an elasticity of demand with respect to co-insurance of 0.37 for home visits by the doctor compared with 0.14 for visits to the doctor (Scitovsky and Snyder, 1972). Similar evidence on the effects of insurance on prescriptions demand is provided from Canada and the UK. Greenlick and Dorsky (1968) found that insurance cover in Ontario, reducing the cost of a prescription to roughly 10 per cent of the average pre-insurance price, led to utilisation by the insured of twice the quantity of prescriptions of the uninsured. This suggests a demand elasticity of 0.4 over the co-insurance range 0.09–1.00. However, this figure may be biased upwards to the extent that the insured are a self-selecting group, choosing insurance because of their worse health. Using UK data from Myers (1972), Phelps and Newhouse examined the demand elasticity of prescriptions. Over the period in question, prices charged by the NHS varied from zero to 12½ pence and so were always relatively low. The implicit co-insurance rate was calculated, from the price charged and the total cost of prescriptions, as between zero and 23 per cent. The fitted demand curve had an elasticity of 0.07, which was similar to that estimated by extrapolation from the Ontario results for the co-insurance range 0–25 per cent. That is, when the cost to the patient of a prescription increases from zero to about 25 per cent of its actual cost, the demand is relatively unresponsive. But if the cost to the patient increases to the full cost of the prescription, the demand responds, according to the Ontario study, to a greater extent. Finally, Friedman (1974) has noted the 6 per cent increase in the quantity of health care consumed by those over sixty-five in the period 1967–71, compared with an increase of 2.4 per cent for those aged nineteen to sixty-four. This followed the introduction of the Medicare programme which meets part of the cost of health care for the old.

None of these estimates suggests that demand is highly elastic in response to co-insurance, but the argument for efficient free (or fully insured) provision would require an elasticity of zero. Therefore, it is possible that insurance leads to inefficiently high consumption of health care, depending on the social benefits of care to the underprivileged, as discussed in Chapter 4. The evidence on insurance effects does not refute any of the demand theories discussed earlier. For a consumer who can make a rational choice, insurance lowers the price of health care and is likely to increase the quantity demanded. For a consumer whose only choice is the yes/no decision of whether to seek health care and to accept the prescribed course of treatment, insurance will increase the amount he will be prepared to pay for relief from a set of symptoms and increase the doctors' knowledge of the amount he is prepared to pay.

5.3.3 Time price effects

Although time prices have been mentioned above, their influence needs more detailed examination. Acton (1975) has developed a model of the demand for medical services that includes time (travel and waiting) as well as conventional money prices. The former have become an increasing proportion of total price paid in America because of the increasing spread of health insurance and the rising opportunity cost of time (wage/income forgone). The predictions of Acton's model were tested on a cross-sectional survey of approximately 2600 users of New York City's 'free' (of user charge) hospital out-patient departments. More specifically, the model emphasises the role of money prices, time prices, earned and unearned income in the demand for medical services. The individual is seen as maximising a utility function U which contains two arguments, medical services h and a composite good X representing all other goods and services. If it requires fixed proportions of money and time to consume both health care and X, and Y is total income, the model can be represented as:

Maximise

$$U = U(h,X) \tag{5.3}$$

subject to

$$(P_h + Wt)h + (P_x + Ws)X \leqslant Y = y + WT \tag{5.4}$$

where

P_h = out-of-pocket money price per unit of medical services;
t = own time input per unit of medical services;
P_x = money price per unit of X;
s = own time input per unit of X;
W = earnings per hour;
y = non-earned income;
T = total amount of time available for market and own production of goods and services.

Acton listed the predictions of the model in response to price changes and income changes. For simplicity, only the former are discussed here. If time is a price, one would expect an own-time price elasticity of demand for medical services that is negative and cross-time price elasticities that are positive. Furthermore, the importance of the former will vary directly with the share of time price in the total price of medical services per unit. Hence, as the out-of-pocket payment for a unit of medical services falls because of the availability of subsidised care or increased insurance cover, the demand becomes relatively more sensitive to time price variations. On this argument the demand for 'free' medical services should be relatively more sensitive to time price changes than the demand for non-free services.

The empirical section of Acton's work is econometrically complex. However, the results support the predictions made above. In particular, the evidence suggests that travel time (as proxied by distance) acts as a price in determining the demand for medical services when free care is available. The results include a negative (own-time price) elasticity of demand of −0.14 which approximates the money price elasticities reported in the literature. For additional material on the role of time in the health care market see Holtman (1972).

5.3.4 *Education effects*

The empirical evidence on the effects of education on the demand for health care is limited and largely inconclusive. Education was found by Grossman to be positively related to health stock, whether it was measured by inference from other data or by days of sickness or restricted activity. But Grossman's results did not yield a statistically significant link between education and the demand for medical care, even though the model predicts a negative relationship because of the enhancement of the effects of gross investment in health by education. Phelps and Newhouse also failed to identify any strong links between education and health care demand, their results being largely insignificant.

5.4 Discussion

All the results surveyed are consistent with the models discussed earlier, in that income and insurance typically exert the expected influences on demand. Therefore, the evidence does not lead us to discard some of the theories and their associated policy prescriptions. However, it is noteworthy that proponents of a particular approach sometimes interpret results in a favourable light by ignoring less sophisticated theoretical explanations. Rosett and Huang, for example, noted that their estimated negative relationship between the ratio of savings to income and expenditure on health care is consistent with the permanent income hypothesis' (i.e. that a high saving-to-income ratio implies a high positive transitory component of income and consumption of health care based on a lower *permanent* income) and also 'with the hypothesis that some part of medical expenditure is treated as investment in household capital' (Rosett and Huang, 1973, p. 289). The latter view accords with Grossman's model, implying choice by individuals between investment in their health and in financial assets. But an equally plausible explanation of the observed relationship requiring a less sophisticated model is that individuals who are taken ill purchase health care from savings as an alternative to reducing current household consumption and run down their savings to finance consumption because of a loss of income during the period of ill health. Of course, this is consistent with the more sophisticated model in that individuals in a market where the treatment of random episodes of ill health is very expensive relative to current income will have an incentive to save as protection against ill health. But this is not to say that they choose to invest in health or other assets, only that they must have a stock of liquid assets to improve their health in the event of illness. The 'choice' to convert liquid assets into health is forced on the consumer by sickness and his doctor's recommended treatment, his only decision being the choice of the maximum amount he is prepared to pay for treatment. This leads us to the evidence that the suppliers of health care are able to increase demand and so appropriate more of the amount the consumer would be prepared to pay in a market system.

5.5 Supplier-induced demand once more

Evans, Parish and Sully (1973) and Evans (1974) have assembled data from various sources that support the view that supplier behaviour in the health care market is responsible for the growth in demand. In particular Evans, Parish and Sully (1973) highlighted the ongoing debate on doctor shortages in Canada which has continued paradoxically during periods of substantial growth in the supply. The evidence broadly suggests that the total workload on all physicians increases when additional practitioners enter an area. The elasticity of this response is of the order of 0.85, indicating that, e.g., 5 per cent more doctors would increase the total workload by over 4 per cent and so reduce workload per physician very little. Such a response may be due to a fall in the time costs of consumers seeking treatment when physician density is higher, but given that time is only one element in the cost of care, this alone is unlikely to account for the response of total workload to physician density.

Evans (1974) cited additional evidence in the form of comparisons of patient-initiated and doctor-initiated contacts. We expect the initial decision to seek treatment to be made by the patient, but we have argued that the doctor will prescribe the treatment and therefore will control the number of repeat visits made by the patient. Canadian data for the period 1957–67 indicated a greater positive correlation between availability and repeat visits than between availability and first-time visits, which does not conflict with the view that increased availability leads to demand generation by increasing repeat visits.

Evans's work also supports earlier studies showing demand elasticities with respect to price of between zero and one. If demand is induced by the supplier, then, subject to the total amount the consumer is prepared to pay, the supplier can control both price and quantity. If the doctor increases his prices he has an incentive to try to offset the fall in demand that might follow for those whose higher priced treatment costs more than their budget by recommending longer or more intensive courses of treatment for those prepared to pay for them. A demand elasticity of less than one might result, but it would not measure the pure price response of demand.

The discussion above suggests that physicians in a market system of health care are generating demand 'needlessly' at the expense of the consumer directly or indirectly through insurance schemes. Certainly there is evidence indicating that rather more operations per head of population at risk are performed in North America than in the UK (see e.g. Vayda, 1973). This is not *prima facie* evidence of demand generation, since it is possible that the UK has too few operations rather than North America too many. But standardisation for the demographic characteristics of the population at risk and the incidence of disease does lead to the implication that it is the US level that is too high.

Excessive surgery may not be due to doctors' attempts to generate revenue. They also face two additional pressures for intervention. The first comes from the patient or his family. Surgery has the appearance of a clear and positive step towards improved health to the layman and so he may insist on surgery because he thinks it will do some good. It is noteworthy that US boys who have been circumcised have an incidence of tonsillectomy seven times greater than those who have not (Bolande, 1969). This is consistent with the view that parents who favour intervention will probably seek it whenever the option is available, even though for both operations the therapeutic benefits are questionable in the great majority of cases. The second pressure is generated by what Fuchs (1968) calls a 'technologic imperative', putting pressure on them to prescribe new, more sophisticated and (frequently by assumption only) more beneficial treatments. This occurs because, particularly where the use of medical techniques to save life is concerned, the technologic imperative effectively removes notions of economic efficiency, concentrating instead on purely technical efficiency. Thus, just as in wartime the cost of the war effort is never counted, so in life-saving any new technique that increases the chance of medical success by even a minute amount is technically preferred regardless of cost. Such innovation is likely to be costly to the patient or his insurance scheme, but in the absence of any clear patient resistance some other control mechanism is required. (For a further discussion of this aspect of supplier behaviour, see Chapters 6 and 11.) Furthermore, while doctors in a state-funded system such as the UK National Health Service have no incentive to generate demand, they may be subject to pressures from producers of other medical inputs, e.g. pharmaceutical companies, to introduce new treatments, not all of which will have proven advantages over the previous treatment method, e.g. tranquillisers. The very large volume of drug advertising to UK doctors certainly supports this. To the extent that career opportunities and status depend on research into new techniques, the pressure to expand the 'demand' for new treatments by prescribing them will remain in a state system. Thus we find, ironically, that similar supplier behaviour might be expected from the most unscrupulous medical practitioner, dedicated to making money, and the most committed, dedicated to improving the health of his patients (recall the discussion of Section 1.3 above).

5.6 The policy implications of demand studies

With policy purposes in mind, the model of demand for health care that comes closest to the reality of consumer choice and is also consistent with all the data on demand is that in which consumers exercise only a yes/no decision, leaving the choice of treatment entirely to the doctor. If doctors, for whatever reasons, are inclined to seek expansion of the demand for health care, a private market without insurance will possibly lead to over-charging and/or the supply of inefficiently large quantities of health care. The introduction of insurance cover will reduce the patients' resistance to demand expansion and so, in the absence of control by the insurance company of both price and quantity, will if anything probably exacerbate excess supply. The implication is that, for efficiency and equity reasons, i.e. to remove tendencies towards excessively high supply and excessive pricing, supervision by the public sector or by an independent third party is required. Note that an insurance company will not necessarily perform such a role.[4] Lower premiums or higher cover are two dimensions on which insurance companies can compete. If the market for insurance favours the latter, e.g. because of consumer fears or willingness to pay premiums for what is perceived as higher quality treatment, then it is easier for the insurance company to lower resistance to demand generation and pass the associated higher costs on to premiums. Supervision by the public sector remains a viable alternative, although clearly, given the scale of the health care sector and the urgency of treatment, only a sample of cases could be vetted. The UK Dental Estimates Board performs this monitoring function, attempting to ensure that dental work paid for jointly by the patient and the NHS is correctly carried out. In addition, pressure for the introduction of new treatments could be countered by insistence on controlled trials (RCTs) of all new techniques to establish their effectiveness independently. At present new drugs are vetted but diagnostic and treatment techniques, e.g. the body scanner and intensive care units for cardiac cases, are not systematically examined before general adoption.

The introduction of such limits on medical behavior would encroach substantially on the doctor's traditional clinical freedom to act in his patient's interests. But if the evidence on demand is accepted, and if no commensurate increase in the effectiveness of treatment can be shown, such encroachment will be in the interests of the patient as the ultimate payer for private, insurance and state-funded health care.

5.7 Summary

As the quotation at the beginning of this chapter and its contents indicate, there remains much empirical (and theoretical) work to be done on the demand for health care. It is apparent that there are many complicating factors that make demand analysis a difficult task, e.g. extensive insurance cover, low or zero money prices, time and trouble costs, etc. The evidence discussed here is mainly American, although work on health care demand has been carried out in the context of the zero user price British National Health Service. The work mainly seeks to relate demand for health care to travel cost variables, i.e. the time and money costs involved. Williams (1977) provides a list of such studies. The final section of this chapter emphasised the strong link between demand and supply in the health care field such that suppliers are in a position to determine demand to a large extent. In the next two chapters supply side factors are brought to the centre of the stage in their own right.

NOTES

1. A lot of the issues discussed here and in the previous chapter are further examined in Chapter 11.

2. As noted in Chapter 1, the double log transformation has the virtue of yielding elasticities directly.
3. The appropriate equation is A.4 in Phelps and Newhouse (1974b).
4. For a more extensive discussion of the role and potential role of the insurance company in the American context and its ability to control health care cost inflation, see the discussion of Havighurst (1977) in Section 11.5.1 below.

REFERENCES

ACTON, J. P. (1975) 'Non-monetary Factors in the Demand for Medical Services: Some Empirical Evidence', *Journal of Political Economy*, Vol. 83, No. 3 (June), pp. 595–614.

AUSTER, R., LEVESON, I. and SARACHEK, D. (1969) 'The Production of Health, an Exploratory Study', *Journal of Human Resources*, Vol. 4, No. 4 (Fall), pp. 412–36; reprinted as Chapter 8, pp. 135–58 in Fuchs, V. R. (ed.) *Essays in the Economics of Health and Medical Care*. New York and London: Columbia University Press for National Bureau of Economic Research.

BOLANDE, R. P. (1969) 'Ritualistic Surgery Circumcision and Tonsillectomy', *New England Journal of Medicine*, Vol. 280, No. 11 (13 March), pp. 591–6.

EVANS, R. G. (1974) 'Supplier-induced Demand; Some Empirical Evidence and Implications', pp. 162–73 in Perlman, M. (ed.), *The Economics of Health and Medical Care*. London and Basingstoke: Macmillan Press for International Economics Association.

EVANS, R. G., PARISH, E. M. A. and SULLY, M. (1973) 'Medical Productivity, Scale Effects and Demand Generation', *Canadian Journal of Economics*, Vol. 6, No. 3 (August), pp. 376–93.

FRIEDMAN, B. (1974) 'A Test of Alternative Demand Shift Responses to the Medicaid Programme', pp. 234–47 in Perlman, M. (ed.), *The Economics of Health and Medical Care*. London and Basingstoke, Macmillan Press for International Economics Association.

FUCHS, V. R. (1968) 'The Growing Demand for Medical Care', *New England Journal of Medicine*, Vol. 279, No. 192 (25 July), pp. 190–5; reprinted as Chapter 4, pp. 61–8 in Fuchs, V. R. (ed.) (1972) *Essays in the Economics of Health and Medical Care*. New York and London: Columbia University Press for National Bureau of Economic Research.

GREENLICK, M. R. and DORSKY, B. J. (1968) 'A Comparison of Drug Utilisation in a Metropolitan Community with Utilisation under Drug Prepayment Plan', *American Journal of Public Health*, Vol. 58, No. 11 (November), pp. 2121–36.

GROSSMAN, M. (1972) *The Demand for Health: A Theoretical and Empirical Investigation* (National Bureau of Economic Research Occasional Paper 119). New York and London: Columbia University Press.

HAVIGHURST, C. C. (1977) 'Controlling Health Care Costs – Strengthening the Private Sector's Hand', *Journal of Health Politics, Policy and Law*, Vol. 1, No. 4 (Winter), pp. 471–98; reprinted as Reprint No. 68, Washington, DC: American Enterprise Institute for Public Policy Research.

HOLTMAN, A. G. (1972), 'Prices, Time and Technology in the Medical Care Market,' *Journal of Human Resources*, Vol. 7, No. 2 (Spring), pp. 179–90.

MYERS, R. J. (1972) *Coverage of Out-of-Hospital Prescriptions under Medicare.* Washington DC: American Enterprise Institute for Public Policy Research.

NEWHOUSE, J. P. (1977) 'Medical Care Expenditure: A Cross-National Survey', *Journal of Human Resources,* Vol. 12, No. 1 (Winter), pp. 115–25.

PHELPS, C. E. and NEWHOUSE, J. P. (1974a) 'Coinsurance, the Price of Time and the Demand for Medical Services', *Review of Economics and Statistics,* Vol. 56, No. 3 (August), pp. 334–42.

PHELPS, C. E. and NEWHOUSE, J. P. (1974b) *Coinsurance and the Demand for Medical Services.* Santa Monica, California: Rand Corporation.

ROSETT, R. N. and HUANG, L. (1973) 'The Effect of Health Insurance on the Demand for Medical Care', *Journal of Political Economy,* Vol. 81, No. 2(1) (March-April), pp. 281–305.

SCITOVSKY, A. A. and SNYDER, A. M. (1972) 'Effects of Coinsurance on Physician Utilisation', *Social Security Bulletin,* Vol. 35, No. 6 (June), pp. 3–19.

VAYDA, E. (1973) 'A Comparison of Surgery Rates in Canada and in England and Wales', *New England Journal of Medicine,* Vol. 289, No. 23 (December), pp. 1224–9.

WILLIAMS, A. (1977) 'What can Economists do to Help Health Service Planning?' pp. 301–35 in ARTIS, N. J. and NOBAY, A. R. (eds) *Studies in Modern Economic Analysis* (Proceedings of the Association of University Teachers of Economics, Edinburgh, 1976). Oxford: Basil Blackwell.

PART III

Health Care Supply Issues

6 The Theory of Supply

> Economists frequently point out our lack of an adequate economic theory of the hospital. Those simple models that have been proposed do not seem to capture the essential institutional details or have great predictive power.
>
> *J. Harris* (1977, p. 467)

6.1 Introduction

In this chapter and the next we review some of the economic models of health care delivery. This literature parallels the conventional theory of the firm but has been developed to examine the divergences in organisation and behaviour of the hospital from the usual theoretical paradigm.[1] We shall emphasise hospitals, giving only a brief discussion of general (or specialist) doctors working outside hospitals, for three reasons. First, hospitals are a more appropriate unit of production for comparison with the 'firm' since they select from a wider range of inputs and are more active producers. (For a general practitioner, own-time is likely to be the dominant input and much of 'production' is achieved passively, within the patient's body, once a course of medication has been recommended.) Second, hospitals are the dominant institutions, in terms of their share of total expenditure, in developed countries and so are an obvious target for detailed economic analysis. Finally, to the extent that they are motivated by similar ends, doctors outside hospitals might be expected to behave in a similar way to hospitals, though with a more limited set of inputs. The reader should also note that the models surveyed below have been developed in the US context. As such they have tended to include various market dimensions such as pricing and demand. To the UK reader more used to the National Health Service, which has virtually no direct charging, this may make such models appear irrelevant. But the basis of the models is a set of general behavioural postulates which can be validly introduced separately from the particular method of payment.

Throughout this chapter we assume that the demand curve, though affected by the quality of the product, is not arbitrarily shifted by supplier behaviour. This is done in order to focus on the other aspects of supply apart from direct influence on demand and is not intended as a negation of earlier discussion.

6.2 The supply of primary care

Before examining the models of hospital behaviour in detail, the operation of the primary care sector warrants some attention, even though it is not our main area of interest, in order to note its similarities with hospitals. When an individual feels ill, but is not faced with a condition requiring immediate treatment, he has to decide a course of action. Doing nothing or treating oneself are probably the most common reactions to illness. But if the illness is serious or prolonged, the individual will consult a supplier of medical care of some kind, be it a factory nurse, a family doctor or specialist. Each will perform a similar task, attempting first to diagnose the patient's illness. Cases that are relatively simple will be treated immediately, while others requiring more complex treatment or diagnostic facilities will be referred to a more specialised 'supplier'. Thus, primary care practitioners act as a filter, allowing only the more serious cases to pass on to the next level of medical care.

Clearly the behaviour of primary suppliers will depend on their objectives, their method of remuneration and the demand of patients for treatment. For example, if doctors are paid a fee for each consultation, then the normal theory of supply and demand would suggest that more doctors will operate in an area where the demand is greater at any given price per consultation. If the price the patient is prepared to pay depends on his income, then demand will be more bouyant in high income areas. Thus in the United States, we find a greater concentration of doctors per head of population in high-income areas. Conversely, if they receive a fee per patient on their lists, doctors lose income by congregating. Only if this is offset by non-monetary rewards (as it may be by, e.g., the environment in holiday resorts) or by monetary rewards from private practice (e.g. in high-income areas) will they be concentrated in particular areas. Thus, the concentration of doctors is less of a problem in the UK than in the USA.

Clearly, a more detailed model of general practice would be required to examine this issue further. However, to the extent that general practice is becoming more complex, e.g. through the introduction of nurses and diagnostic equipment, models of hospital behaviour may be relevant for the general practitioner. Each type of supplier of health care takes a similar kind of decision, assessing patients, deciding on a course of treatment and separating those whose treatment will help maximise the supplier's objectives from those whose treatment will not. As we shall discuss below, the nature of these objectives is crucial to the outcome.

6.3 The supply of hospital care

Theories of hospital activity face three particular problems in seeking a rigorous and fruitful analysis of the supply of health care. These concern the choice of decision-maker, the market environment and the quality of care. After considering each of these, we turn to the models themselves.

Given the importance of charitable and religious foundations in the history of hospital care and their continuing major role in the non-governmental hospital sector, the main behavioural assumption is that the hospital is not profit-seeking. However, this restriction is subsequently removed for a comparison of profit and non-profit-making hospital behaviour. Then after the discussion of each type of model we examine the empirical evidence concerning the models' predictions and their implications for efficiency and equity.

6.3.1 *Whose maximand?*

The traditional theory of the firm focuses on the profit-maximising entrepreneur who controls the choice of inputs and outputs and reaps profits as a residue in excess of other costs. The introduction of managers separate from owners will alter this framework since maximum profit for the owner may not maximise the objective function of the manager. He may prefer to divert some potential profit into providing improved offices, more skilled or attractive staff, etc. (see Williamson, 1963).

For the hospital, responsibility for decision-making may depend not only on administrative managers but also on four other groups: doctors (and nurses), trustees (for non-profit-making hospitals), trade unionists and politicians. Each group may be pursuing different objectives and so the assumption of a single 'hospital' decision in the models that follow is misleading. Action in response to any particular stimulus may represent an *ad hoc* compromise rather than a negotiated agreement on objectives, and so each model is likely to fit reality only to a limited degree if it subsumes possible conflicts between objectives.

Doctors in particular are in an unusual position compared to other 'production' workers. In the conventional firm, a decision on input combinations and output rates taken by management is handed down the organisational pyramid to the shop floor. Obviously, unions and management may negotiate over details, but ultimately a decision, effectively removing or constraining the individual production worker's choice, is arrived at. Budgetary and purchasing decisions can then be made higher up the organisation in the knowledge that x workers will use y components and z machines per month.

Now consider the doctor. Although he is the main direct producer (a surgeon is, after all, a highly skilled manual worker), he uses considerable individual discretion in choosing the inputs that will achieve the ultimate output, an improvement in patient health. This choice will depend on his diagnosis and his objective function and so need not be the same for all doctors faced with a given case. (Variations in behaviour of doctors can lead to major differences in the health care provided. See Cooper (1975, Chapter 6) and also Chapter 10 below for a discussion of this aspect of the UK National Health Service.) In addition, many of the resource inputs at the doctor's disposal will be shared by colleagues with competing demands for their use. Resolution of conflict is clearly achieved somehow but, although the mechanism is not necessarily efficient, it has been examined very little. In view of the large expenditures that may be involved, e.g. in the choice of more expensive alternative drugs of little additional usefulness, further research is required.

The remaining three groups, though less dominant than the doctor, also influence hospital decision-making directly or indirectly. Trustees of non-profit hospitals may seek objectives such as prestige by the purchase of sophisticated capital equipment or the hiring of highly qualified staff. Trade unions, aside from exercising political pressure on elected representatives, may influence the choice of inputs directly if these affect the jobs or conditions of employment of their members. And politicians, though typically aloof from the general decision-making of the hospital, may sometimes intervene directly to secure a particular change in hospital activity (e.g. the moratorium imposed by the UK Department of Health on heart transplant operations in Britain).

In view of the multiplicity of decision-makers (a complication that we do not propose to resolve here), the models discussed below must be viewed (more than most) as abstractions from reality. Each of the early models takes the hospital or its medical staff as the sole decision-maker, ignoring conflicts between and within different groups. But to the extent that the models adopt a plausible set of objectives and produce general conclusions of a qualitative kind, they are of interest.

6.3.2 *The competitive environment*

We have noted earlier in this book how consumer ignorance may effectively give the producers of health care a monopoly advantage. The consumer is no longer readily able to judge the quality of the product and so focuses instead on some proxy indicator (e.g. the age and equipment of a hospital or the letters after a doctor's name). The effect of this will be to encourage, in a competitive environment, the use of a similar, high-quality mix of inputs by all hospitals. Thus competition may, uncharacteristically, increase costs rather than the reverse. In addition, where non-profit-making and profit-making hospitals operate in the same area, the normal competitive outcome will not occur because of the absence of profits in one part of the market and its possible effects on pricing and supply. As we shall see, the problems raised by this interaction are not wholly resolved by the models that attempt to do so. Finally, the competitive environment is also affected by the cost structure of hospitals. The construction cost of a hospital, particularly one equipped to modern standards and supplying high-quality care, is extremely high, e.g. £20,000 per bed (Culyer and Cullis, 1974) and the cost of care declines with utilisation. Thus, hospitals are natural monopolies and local competition will be weak (see Section 2.3.3 above).

6.3.3 The quality of care supplied

Aside from its effects on the competitive environment, quality may also be important for the producer *per se*. A doctor committed by the Hippocratic Oath to doing as much as possible for his patient is likely, in the absence of cost constraints, to try to achieve the highest quality of care. The precise meaning of the term 'quality' is difficult to specify beyond this simple hypothesis of medical behaviour. Giving the patient the 'best' care may imply giving the treatment with the highest *quantity* of inputs if quality is associated with higher cost. Therefore, in the discussion that follows, the quantity of care will refer to the number of cases treated and the quality of care to the type of treatment as seen by patients or doctors. Given inbuilt medical preferences for quality, more resources will be taken up by the doctor for treatment whenever the constraints permit. More significantly, the fixity of capital, which places a top limit on the quantity of cases that can be treated, will encourage the use of current revenue to increase quality, as will advancing medical technology. Therefore, quality becomes a dominant issue in all the models that follow. Although none of these is wholly integrated with a theory of demand, each assumes a demand structure in which quality is of key importance.

6.4 A theory of non-profit-making hospital behaviour

A model of effects of non-profit-making objectives on the provision of medical services has been developed in detail by Newhouse (1970). The decision-makers of the hospital are assumed to have two objectives which they seek to maximise: the quantity of care delivered, and its quality. The first objective is clearly uncontroversial. Since the aim of a charity hospital is to reduce the suffering owing to ill health, it requires only the assumption that more care leads to improved health for the quantity of care to be an objective. Quality of care is assumed to be an objective in addition to quantity because of the key role of quality in medical services. Newhouse links the quality of care to the prestige of hospital staff which itself replaces profits as a target for the decision-maker. Furthermore, as we have discussed in Chapter 4 above, the quality of care is likely to be of great significance to the consumer. Thus Newhouse assumes that the demand curve for care shifts up as quality rises, though this is not a feature that is readily integrated with existing demand theory. Figure 6.1 shows the possible equilibria for the hospital. Care of increasing quality (q_i, $i=0, 1, 2, 3$) can be provided at an average cost per unit shown by the associated average cost curve AC_i. (The absence

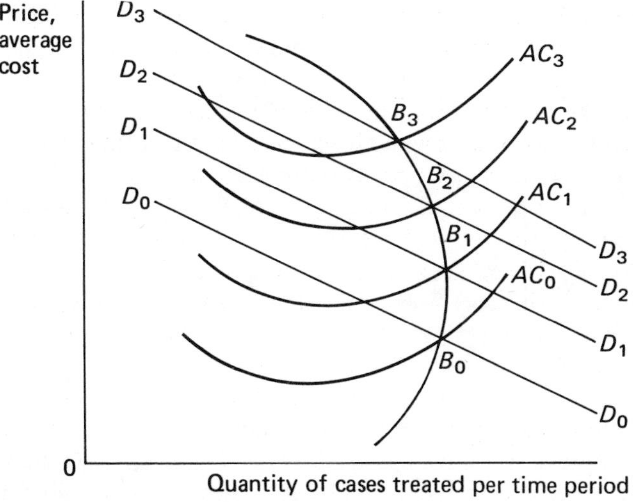

Figure 6.1 Demand and average cost at various levels of quality

of marginal cost reflects the non-profit-making motive. Patient payments need only cover average cost so that the hospital breaks even.) For a charitable foundation the costs to be covered by charges may be less than the total cost of provision, the deficiency being made up from the charity's funds.

Associated with each quality level is a demand curve D_iD_i which, together with the cost curve, gives the break-even quantity of care of any given quality level. If we identify a series of these break-even points B_i for each quality level, we can construct a transformation curve showing the possible combinations of quantity and quality that the hospital can attain. A key assumption in its construction is that beyond some quality level the cost of further increases in quality rises more rapidly than the demand for care. That is, when quality is high already, consumers attach less importance to a further increase in quality (declining marginal utility) but the cost of raising quality further is increasing (increasing marginal cost of quality).[2] As a result of the assumed behaviour of demand and cost this curve is backward-bending in Figure 6.2 below.

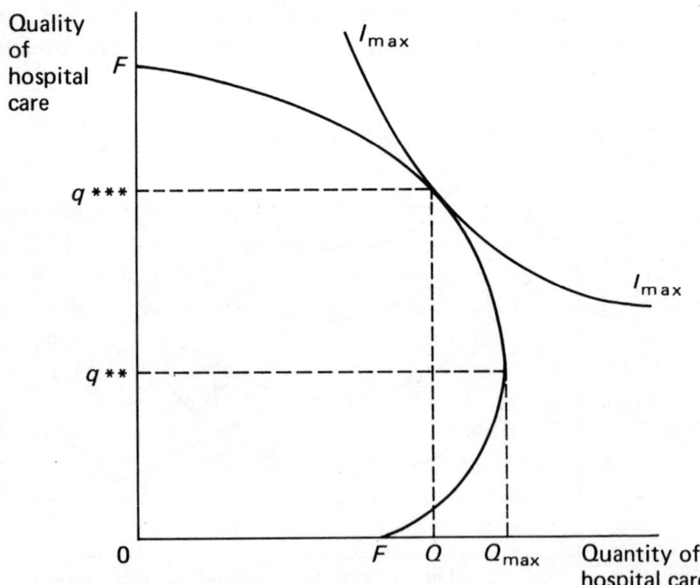

Figure 6.2 The optimal quality–quantity combination

The decision-maker then chooses the optimal levels of quality and quantity by selecting the combination on the possibility frontier *FF* that gives him the highest level of utility; graphically a typical tangency between the possibility frontier and highest attainable indifference curve, I_{max}. This shows that, with the indifference map postulated, he chooses three-star quality and a quantity of output (i.e. patients treated or patient days of care) Q that is lower than the maximun Q_{max}. Clearly, with the right indifference map, quantity Q_{max} and two-star quality could be selected. But at the point that the transformation curve turns back on itself, its slope is vertical. Thus, an indifference curve will be tangential at that point only if it has a vertical slope. Yet this would imply that the marginal utility of quality to the decision-maker is zero, which violates our initial assumption that both quality and quantity yielded utility to the decision-maker (and by implication from consumer theory, that he can never be satiated (marginal utility = 0) with either). Therefore, a solution to the left of Q_{max} is inevitable as long as the decision-maker always attaches some positive marginal utility to the quality of care. The implications of this quality emphasis are discussed below.

6.5 Hospital activity in a public system

Newhouse specifically examines charitable hospitals but his argument can also apply to publicly financed hospitals in the UK. The major difference is that public hospitals in the British National Health Service face no effective competition for the majority of their cases. Thus, the demand for their services is likely to be much less sensitive to the quality of care offered. They also receive a fixed budget and do not recoup any revenue from patients. Therefore the trade-off curve between quantity and quality is different in shape from that depicted earlier. Increases in quality are always associated with reductions in quantity because of the fixed budget. The choice of quality and quantity by the medical decision-makers will reflect their objective function. However, given the likely importance of the 'technologic imperative' discussed earlier, the quality of care is likely to be higher than the minimum and the quantity of cases treated lower than the maximum. Higher quality in this situation is not necessarily undesirable in that it may increase the probability of successful treatment at the expense of treating fewer cases. But such is the emphasis on quality in medicine that new higher-quality inputs are frequently adopted as minimum requirements without detailed evaluation of the contribution they make. Hence the behaviour of a public hospital system may be to the benefit of the patients receiving care for diseases causing death but may lead to fewer cases of these or of other less serious kinds being treated. The political and social sensitivity of life-saving treatments makes any movement away from high-quality care for these risks extremely difficult even where the benefits of such care are not demonstrable.

6.6 The hospital as conspicuous producer

Lee (1971) has presented a model based on interdependent hospital behaviour. This model is similar to Newhouse's in that it focuses on the key role of the quality of care in influencing decision-makers and consumers. The single decision-maker of the hospital is seen as a utility-maximiser whose utility is determined by such factors as salary, prestige and job satisfaction. These and other relevant influences on utility are assumed to depend on the 'status' of the hospital. Each hospital manager has a target status and seeks to minimise the gap between target and actual status. But status, much like quality, is not readily measurable and is associated by Lee with a set of desired inputs of staff and equipment. Hospitals attempt to achieve a similar status to those around them since this raises the utility of the manager directly through the improvement of facilities and indirectly through the attraction of high-status medical and technical staff by such facilities. Patients are again charged a price that covers the total cost of the hospital rather than the cost of their care, in Lee's model. Therefore, the ability of the hospital decision-maker to pursue his status goal requires that patients are prepared to meet the higher costs of higher-quality inputs and that consumers behave as in the Newhouse model.

The result of the pursuit of quality in either model is that, in order to be seen by consumers to be as good as surrounding hospitals, each hospital will equip itself to deal with a wide range of conditions in the most sophisticated way consistent with costs and revenue. Thus, as Lee emphasised, available capacity for treatments such as heart surgery is greatly in excess of the efficient amount since facilities and skills are used infrequently, losing the smoothing effect of practice (see Table 6.1). This is a more

Table 6.1 Available Capacity for Heart Surgery

Type of procedure	Number of hospitals reporting facilities	Percentage with *x* cases per year 0	1–9	10–49	50+	Not known
Open-heart	327	11	30	36	17	6
Closed-heart	777	30	43	18	6	4

Source: Quoted by Lee (1971) from Spencer and Eiseman (1965)

serious difficulty than the question of general quality discussed earlier. If the quality of non-capital inputs is higher, it may make some contribution to patients' health that justifies the higher price. But if all patients are paying for high-quality–high-cost capital equipment which is of benefit to only a few patients, who presumably would be unable to pay the full cost of these facilities themselves, then many patients are needlessly paying a high price to maintain the excess supply of sophisticated capital, even though they are prepared to pay this high price for care. We examine this question in more detail below.

The extent of underuse is highlighted by comparison of Table 6.1 with the view of a leading American cardiac specialist that one surgical performance per week is required to maintain surgical skills (quoted by Lee). Presumably many more cases per week would be required to achieve minimum average cost.

To summarise, quality is assumed to be of paramount importance to non-profit-making behaviour and this is shown to lead to higher quality of care in terms of resource inputs though the quality of the output – health improvements – is unknown. Excess capacity of sophisticated capital equipment is simply another dimension of quality, but it may be a more serious one, given the likely high cost and underuse of such facilities. Thus, the problem facing the government is whether to intervene in the market in order to control the zeal for quality and increase social welfare. Examples of such intervention can now be found in the USA e.g. the recent restrictions on the purchase of body-scanners requiring prior demonstration of a local need for additional units.

6.7 The effects of quality bias

In the models above the quality of health care is of prime importance. This reflects a widely held view among health economists that the nature of health care as a commodity makes quality a major focus of attention for both consumer and producer. In other economic areas, the quality of the product is clearly relevant but receives little emphasis. If the consumer finds that a baker sells him stale bread or a film director sells him stale dialogue, he suffers no permanent loss. In future, he can avoid both suppliers and so improve the quality of consumption. Now consider health care. The bad product may be fatal. This alone will encourage the consumer to seek licensing and professional standards for doctors for his own protection. Even if he survives inferior treatment, the effects can easily be permanent. A malpractice suit against his doctor may well provide some compensation, but it is questionable whether sums of money can wholly replace the unnecessary loss of a large sub-set of possible social and work activities. And in the absence of compensation, 'being wise after the event' and 'shopping elsewhere in future', the conventional responses, are of little use.

Whether it is bread, films or health care that is being supplied, however, the threat of withdrawal by the consumer will give an incentive to producers to maintain a satisfactory product quality.

A further difficulty arises, however, if the consumer or the economist is unable to measure the quality of care he has received (e.g. because of the problems of consumer ignorance discussed earlier). The taste of bread and the entertainment value of a film are both immediately recognisable to the consumer. Thus, he knows when each good has failed to meet his accustomed standard. But for health care, the consumer has little or no clear knowledge of how he should feel after treatment if he has received the best quality care rather than something less. Comparable repeat trials are frequently impossible and the process of obtaining information from other consumers is difficult. Therefore, if quality is a prime mover for the consumer, he must find a proxy measure of quality by which to make his consumption decisions. This is likely to be the quality of the inputs used by the hospital which is in turn reflected in costs and prices.

Although framed in terms of consumers, this discussion is central to the theory of supplier behaviour. If the consumer prefers a higher quality of care then the supplier who wishes to continue to treat patients in a competitive environment must meet these preferences. More particularly, if high-quality inputs have little or no effect on patient health but merely serve as a magnet with which to attract patients (e.g. underused heart surgery units), it is tempting to conclude that a misallocation of resources to quality is occurring. Patients are paying a higher price than necessary for care that only seems to be better. Furthermore, as we shall discuss later, quality bias is also likely to occur in profit-making hospitals because of the effects on demand and so, although their higher cost of capital may reduce the extent of excess capacity in profit-making hospitals, it will not necessarily be removed by the familiar competitive pressures.

However, even the excess capacity of heart surgery facilities is not necessarily undesirable, in terms of its contribution to social welfare – defined loosely as the wellbeing of the individuals in society. Thus, Lee (1971) talks of the 'welfare loss to consumers' from the emphasis on quality misleadingly. It is the preference of consumers for high-quality care that permits the emphasis on quality. Doctors may have a built-in prejudice for quality as part of their training, and their willingness to prescribe high-quality care may be increased by the knowledge that a patient has insurance cover. But the costs of any resulting excessive high quality cannot simply be termed a loss of social welfare. In the last resort, if a consumer judges himself to be better off when receiving what he perceives as higher-quality care, then he suffers no welfare loss when purchasing it. Thus, the conventional welfare economics argument is that, if consumers prefer a higher quality of care and are prepared to pay for it, there is no reason to prevent them receiving it.

Of course, this result highlights a major weakness of welfare economics in tackling an issue such as this. Social welfare depends on individual welfare, and so if individuals believe themselves to be better off with high-quality resources used for their health care, then social welfare is also greater. An alternative approach is to introduce an 'ethical observer', essentially someone who can recommend intervention in the market place if he judges that resources are not being allocated so as to maximise social welfare. Typically this role is fulfilled by the government. Thus, the government might justify intervention to prevent excess capacity and unnecessarily high-quality inputs on the grounds that it knows better than the consumer the effects of his consumption upon himself and seeks to protect him from himself (a merit want). This is a major reason for policies to protect children but also leads to restrictions on the behaviour of adults (e.g., drug consumption is legislated against not only because of possible externalities but to save the addict from himself). Clearly, the extent to which the reader accepts individual preferences as the basis for the allocation of resources will determine his acceptance or rejection of the ethical observer approach. However, it is a useful method of focusing attention on an alternative perspective and so we retain it in subsequent discussion. A further justification for intervention can be provided aside from the ethical observer's view about what is 'best' for society. If health care can be sensibly consumed only in large indivisible amounts (e.g., half a course of treatment may well be useless), then quality bias which raises the price paid by consumers may prevent the poor consuming any health care. Thus, quality bias can be opposed on equity grounds also.

Government licensing of hospital facilities would remove excess capacity if the number of licensed beds was determined by criteria of operating efficiency rather than consumer willingness to pay. But decisions on the quality of inputs would be much less easy to restrict because it would be more difficult to measure their quality and decide on technical grounds that certain inputs were ineffective in changing the patient's health in comparison with cheaper alternatives. This is particularly so where life-saving treatments are introduced because they are thought to increase the *probability* of saving life, even when the anticipated increase in probability is small. Where this has been shown (Mather *et al.*, 1971) the policy response may be equally difficult to implement. As noted in Chapter 1, Mather's results questioned the effectiveness of intensive care (as compared with bed-rest at home) for patients recovering from heart attack. Even if these results were accepted widely, it is difficult to imagine an elected representative challenging the medical establishment by attempting to reduce the provision of such facilities. Equally, it is hard to see the public taking sides with politicians against doctors.

An extension of intervention to the supply of all, or most, health care seems more likely to limit the 'misallocation' of resources into high-quality inputs. Hospitals in the UK National Health Service are not competing directly for patients and so input quality improvements in one hospital are less likely to be repeated across many, particularly as there is a central authority to oversee and prevent excess capacity. But if health care decision-makers *in any environment* share the view that input quality is to be pursued as a means of improving the quality of outcomes, we might expect even in a national health service to find that a wide range of inputs are of higher quality and cost but of no proven impact on outcome. As a result, the whole service might be over-expanded relative to other areas of public expenditure where evaluation is more feasible. (For some challenging arguments on the role of medical technological improvements on health see, e.g., Illich, 1976; Cochrane, 1972.)

However, it is important to bear in mind the fundamental issue that the relationship between quality of inputs and quality of outcome is not a clearly measurable one. The approach above and its conclusions about misallocation rest on the assumption that input quality is a poor indicator of the quality of care and health improvement. If this assumption is mistaken, and, as Jacobs (1974) pointed out in his survey of hospital models, if there is no usable definition of quality in models of hospital behaviour, then it is impossible to prove that quality has changed or that resources have indeed been misallocated. As we shall see further in the next chapter, such measurement problems are a major difficulty confronting the health economist.

6.8 Profit-making and non-profit-making hospitals

So far, we have said very little about the market environment and the effects of non-profit-making hospital emphasis on quality on the profit-making sector of the market. Essentially, they face a dilemma. If they are to compete for consumers with the non-profit-making sector, then, if quality is of paramount importance to the consumers, the profit-seeking hospitals must offer a comparable quality of care. But if they are to compete with the charges of non-profit-making hospitals, then they too will make no profits and will cease to trade. Therefore, it is interesting to consider how profit-making hospitals survive in a market where non-profit-making hospitals are a common feature. (Even in the UK profit-making nursing homes providing care for a particular group of patients – the elderly – are common.)

Clearly, if the non-profit-making hospital sector(s) cannot provide for all the demands for medical services at a break-even price (or zero price for public health services), then a fraction of demand is unmet. Alternatively, if non-profit-making health services are priced to cover total cost (minus any subsidies received) they may be reluctant to respond to excess demand by raising prices even though the quasi-profits made could be used to increase the future supply of facilities. As a result, some demand will be unmet and again will encourage a profit-making sector. But there may be significant differences in the type of demand that the profit-making sector seeks to treat and in the methods used to treat it.

A very clear exposition of the possible differences has been provided by Schweitzer and Rafferty (1976) in their comparative analysis of the two sectors in the United States. Their approach requires us to make a number of simplifying assumptions, but these do not have a fundamental impact on the outcome of their comparisons.

(a) We consider only two diseases, one of which requires more capital-intensive methods of treatment than the other, e.g. surgical and medical specialties.

(b) The production function relating inputs of labour and capital to the output of numbers of cases is homogeneous of degree 1; i.e., constant returns to scale exist.

From these two assumptions we can construct isoquants for

each disease, showing the inputs of labour and capital required to treat a given number of such cases – k_i k_i for the capital-intensive disease, l_i l_i for the labour intensive in Figure 6.3.

To these isoquants we can add an iso-cost line showing the different combinations of labour and capital that can be obtained from a given budget. These iso-cost lines differ for the two kinds of hospital, reflecting the further assumption that there are differences in the cost of capital for each. Non-profit-making hospitals are argued to have access to funds for capital equipment without incurring any cost, from donations by the public. Alternatively there are various subsidies or tax concessions to non-profit-making organisations which artificially lower the cost of capital. Furthermore, as our earlier models suggested, the pursuit of quality may lead to more sophisticated capital being employed by non-profit-making hospitals because such capital contributes to increased utility or status for the hospital decision-maker who gains no financial reward from acting more efficiently. Conversely, the profit-seeking hospital has to obtain its capital at the going capital–market rate of interest, and its decision-maker will have less discretion on investment. (However, if non-profit-making hospitals use

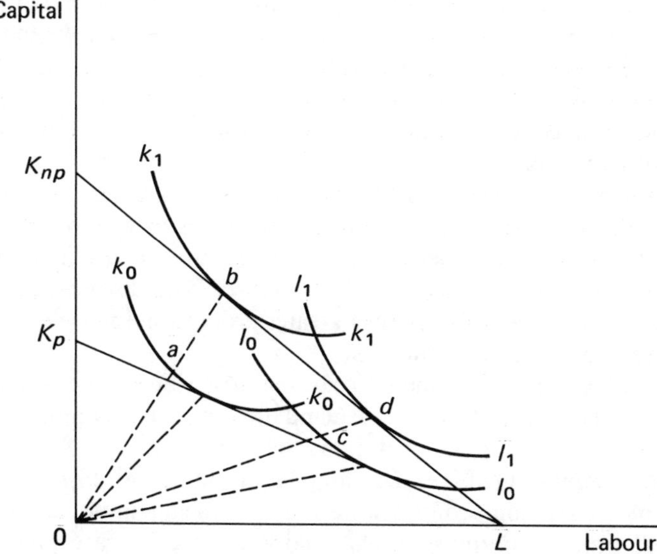

Figure 6.3 Choice of input mixes for profit and non-profit-making hospitals

donations and tax concessions to subsidise all inputs, the model effectively collapses.)

Therefore, although both types of hospital have the same production technology, they are assumed to have different costs. The non-profit-making hospital in Figure 6.3 has iso-cost line LK_{np} and the profit-seeking hospital has iso-cost line LK_p. For any given quantity of either case type, we would expect to find that the profit-seeking hospital would use a lower capital-to-labour ratio for treatment (as shown by the rays from the origin to the tangency points). Also for a given cost constraint, the higher cost of capital for the profit-seeking hospital restricts it to treating a smaller number of cases of either type, but the reduction in cases treated is greater if the hospital treats only the capital-intensive disease than if it treats only the labour-intensive one. (This result comes directly from the assumption that the production functions relating inputs to numbers of cases treated were homogeneous of degree 1. The ratio of cases treated by the profit-seeker to cases treated by the non-profit-making hospital is found by taking a ray from the origin and finding the ratios Oa/Ob and Oc/Od. Constant returns to scale ensure that these are the ratios of the quantities associated with each isoquant.)

From the isoquant diagram above Schweitzer and Rafferty construct the average cost curves for the two diseases, k and l, and the two hospitals, np and p (Figure 6.4).

Long-run average cost per case is constant over all levels of output and equal to marginal cost because of the assumption of constant returns. The lower cost of capital for the non-profit-making hospital leads to a lower average cost per case for both diseases, AC_{knp} and AC_{lnp}. But because of the effects of capital intensity on the number of cases treated by the profit-seeking hospital, its average costs, though higher for both diseases, exceed the non-profit-making costs by a greater proportion for the capital-intensive disease, AC_{kp} and AC_{knp}.

So far we have considered only the cost side of the market. We can now introduce the demand for care to examine price and output effects. Figure 6.4 shows the demand curves of patients for the capital-intensive (D_k) and labour-intensive (D_l) disease treatments. A non-profit-making hospital facing these demands would produce outputs of Q_{knp} and Q_{lnp} of each case type. A profit-seeking hospital, on the other hand, would produce lower

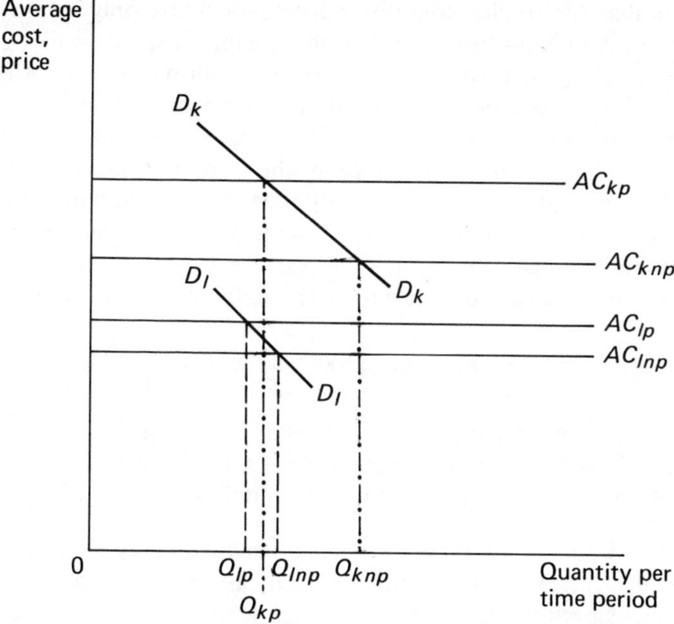

Figure 6.4 Output levels for profit and non-profit-making hospitals

outputs of both types of case, but, given the demand curves shown, would treat proportionately fewer cases of the capital-intensive disease and more cases of the labour-intensive disease. Therefore, Schweitzer and Rafferty conclude with the prediction that, when faced with similar demands, profit-seeking hospitals will treat a less capital-intensive case-mix than non-profit-making hospitals.[3]

We will return to the operation of this model below. First we consider the evidence that bears on the prediction of the model. The obvious characteristic of profit-seeking hospitals assumed in the initial discussion of the model is that these hospitals face a higher cost of capital. This distorts their iso-cost curve and, as a result, for a given quantity of care they will use a lower capital-to-labour ratio. Tests on this aspect of the model face substantial difficulties both in identifying similar cases in different types of hospital and also in estimating the capital intensity of their treatment in each hospital. Schweitzer and Rafferty produce data on this aspect of the model but are obliged to stress that the results, confirming their model, are only tentative.

The major conclusion, that profit-seeking hospitals will treat a less-capital intensive mix of cases, is confirmed in two ways. First, if it is assumed that the mean length of stay in hospital of patients with a given disorder is an indicator of the patients' use of capital equipment (since if they are not using it they could be nursed outside the hospital), then the profit-seeking hospital would be expected to treat a greater proportion of shorter-stay cases than longer-stay ones. This can be tested by calculating a weighted measure of case mix and length of stay of the form:

$$I = \sum_{d=1}^{n} R_{id} LOS_d \,.\, (100) \left(\sum_{d=1}^{n} R_d LOS_d \right)^{-1}$$

where R_{id} = proportion of cases of type d in hospital i;
R_d = proportion of cases of type d in all hospitals;
LOS_d = mean length of stay in hospital of all cases of type d.

This measure compares the mean length of stay that would exist in a hospital if its patients in each case type had the sample average length of stay with the average length of stay of patients in the whole sample. If a hospital has a mix of cases biased towards shorter-stay cases, then its estimated mean length of patient stay when each patient is assumed to stay the average number of days for his disease will be less than the sample average stay. The index thus calculates estimated stay as a percentage of the sample mean stay, with figures below 100 per cent indicating a bias towards shorter-stay.

The proprietary hospitals in their sample were found by Schweitzer and Rafferty to have an index of 81.9 compared with a range of 97.9 to 106.8 for the voluntary hospitals. This confirms their hypothesis that the proprietary hospitals adopt a shorter-stay case mix. This finding is similar to their finding on the capital intensity of treatment, where case proportions were weighted by average expenditure on laboratory and radiological services instead of by average length of stay. The case mix of proprietary hospitals was such that, had they spent the average amount for each case type of these services, they would have a mean expenditure per case of 81.1 per cent of the figure for all case types. Thus, if length of stay and use of laboratory and radiological services are a satisfactory proxy for the capital intensity of particular disease treatment, the Schweitzer and Rafferty hypothesis is confirmed. However it cannot be accepted unreservedly given the small sample (sixty-three New England hospitals, of which only four are proprietary), the assumed (rather than established) links between capital intensity, length of stay and laboratory services, and the likely incentives for profit-making hospitals to seek a rapid turnover of cases for higher profits.

Further evidence of behavioural differences between the two sectors of hospital care is provided by Clarkson (1972). He has argued that the absence of a profit-maximising objective in non-profit-making hospitals will lead to differences in behaviour. In particular, market information is likely to be less effectively collected and used by non-profit-making hospital decision-makers because of its reduced importance. Thus, Clarkson hypothesises that non-profit-making hospitals will be more out of step with the markets in which they purchase inputs than proprietary hospitals seeking profits.

The evidence produced in support of this hypothesis shows that it is broadly confirmed; e.g., a greater proportion of non-profit-making hospitals were shown to give automatic salary increases to staff, and the non-profit-making hospitals showed greater variation in the wages paid to a wide range of staff.

Similar behaviour is suggested also by the evidence of high profit margins on tranquillisers sold in the UK National Health Service (Monopolies Commission, 1973). The absence of a profit motive is likely to weaken the pressure exerted by negotiators when purchasing such drugs and to lead to overcharging. Similarly, since costs do not impinge on the individual doctor in the National Health Service (and to some degree in all hospitals), drug prices are not known to doctors who have no incentive to find them out (unless their activities are audited) and choose cheaper substitutes. (For evidence relating to this issue see for example, Skipper *et al.*, 1976).

6.9 The effects of 'skimming'

If profit-making hospitals 'skim' off a particular type of case, or at least generally operate with a higher proportion of less capital-intensive cases, we can examine whether this behaviour is undesirable. However, before attempting to resolve its desirability, we can consider the market environment, which permits the skimming of cases by the profit-making sector. In particular we need to consider the demand for treatment in profit-making hospitals.

We have established above that the average costs to be covered by revenue from patients will be higher than for profit-making hospitals. (In the UK context, National Health Service hospitals make no charge at all since all their costs are covered by government funds.) Thus, there will be a demand for the higher priced care only if it is providing not only health care of equal quality but also a service that the consumer regards as worth paying an extra amount for. Two reasons why this might be the case are as follows.

(a) If the quality of treatment in its medical and 'hotel' (i.e. room, meals, etc.) dimensions is perceived by consumers to be higher in the profit-seeking hospital, then they may be prepared to pay an additional sum for treatment there.

(b) If treatment of acceptable quality is available *immediately* in profit-seeking hospitals, then consumers may be prepared to pay for immediate treatment to avoid prolongation of pain and disability.

The latter reason may be particularly significant in the UK, where the cost of treatment (for the uninsured) in profit-seeking institutions such as private hospitals and nursing homes may be substantial by comparison with the NHS (though no systematic data on the costs of care of various kinds in profit-seeking and non-profit-making institutions in the private sector of UK medicine exist at present). However, cost will be less important in any private systems where the patient's costs are covered by insurance.

More important, the latter reason may bear a systematic relationship to the capital intensity of treatment. Let us first of all make a plausible simplifying assumption: that capital intensity of treatment for surgical cases is correlated positively with their urgency; i.e., that emergency surgery requires more capital per case than so-called 'cold' surgery for conditions that do not endanger life. Typically, emergencies receive immediate care while cold surgery cases are deferred. Thus it will be patients requiring less capital-intensive treatment who are on waiting lists, and it will be these patients whom the profit-seeking hospitals will be best equipped to treat. Thus, the provision of a less capital-intensive sector increases the efficiency of the health care system by matching up the capital–labour mix with the appropriate case types and reducing the extent of surplus capacity that would arise from the capital price distortion if less capital-intensive cases were treated in a more capital-intensive hospital. Of course, any such improvement in efficiency may be offset in the view of the governmental decision-maker if it also leads to inequality in treatment between high-income groups who can afford higher cost care and low-income groups who cannot.

Casual observers of the UK health care institutions may feel that the analysis so far fits more closely the American context, in which it was originally developed by Schweitzer and Rafferty, since in the UK much of the treatment provided outside the National Health Service is carried out in non-profit-making hospitals which recoup their costs through insurance cover or charges on patients. But this overlooks the large number of privately owned homes that provide care for old people. Medically, such cases require a relatively low capital intensity of treatment, and so their location in proprietary institutions accords with the model presented earlier. The cost of capital is zero to the NHS hospital itself, is subsidised by fund-raising and charitable status for the non-profit-making sector and is unsubsidised only for the profit-seeking institutions. Thus we would expect, and indeed would find, capital intensity varying with the cost of capital. The desirability of profit-making hospitals (and nursing homes, etc.) and in particular the effects of skimming have been a feature of recent debate in the UK on the existence of private practice within the National Health Service. However, here we wish to concentrate on the general welfare implications, leaving aside detailed consideration of the institutional context.

We have noted that one advantage derived from the skimming behaviour of profit-making hospitals is greater efficiency in the provision of care. Capital-intensive cases are treated in the non-profit-making sector where capital is under-priced, while labour-intensive cases are treated in the profit-making sector. If, in the absence of profit-making hospitals, non-profit-making hospitals undertook to treat all cases, then some of these cases would be underusing the specialised (capital and labour skills) of non-profit-making hospitals. Efficiency would be increased if all hospitals treated the cases appropriate for their capital and labour, particularly if non-profit hospitals pursue higher input quality for its own sake.

But this is too simple an argument! Facilities in advanced acute hospitals may be underused if the hospital's beds are occupied by geriatric patients. Yet there is nothing to prevent non-profit-making institutions setting up less capital-intensive treatment units to provide care of this kind also. Thus, skimming is likely to occur because non-profit-making hospitals cannot or do not attempt to treat all sickness. Some demand will always be unmet if non-profit-making hospitals do not raise prices when faced with excess demand, or if demand is inelastic. The creation of profit-making institutions is the inevitable market response, e.g., the large number of rest homes for the elderly in the UK is a reflection of the inability of the National Health Service, with its fixed number of beds, to accommodate every such patient while also treating the acute cases arising from the rest of the population.

The question of our ethical observer or government examining the effects of profit-making activity resolves itself into a question of meeting the demand while ameliorating any inequalities regarded as undesirable. If, as we have suggested, the profit-making sector supplies some of the demand that charity or the tax-financed public hospitals are unwilling or unable to meet, then there can be no objection to it. However, if the profit-making sector does not merely treat unmet demand but also changes the pattern of cases treated, it may be less desirable. This can occur if the profit-making institutions do not increase the supply of those resources that are constraining the delivery of care. For example, if profit-making hospitals are able to bid doctors and nurses away from the non-profit-making sector, then they may treat more of the labour-intensive sector. Thus the proprietary sector may not only skim cases but may also alter the overall pattern of cases treated towards a higher proportion of less acute cases.

However, this conclusion is by no means unambiguous. The ultimate outcome will depend on insurance cover, unmet demand, the elasticity of demand and the supply of resources. The simplest test of the welfare effects of profit-making hospitals is to examine whether they increase the supply of resources to meet demands for health care. Beyond this, their effects require a more detailed analysis than has so far emerged in the literature.

6.10 Two firms in one!

The final model considered here is contained in a recent paper by Harris (1977), who discussed the nature of the internal organisation of hospitals. Harris hoped that future hospital models would face directly questions of internal conflict resolution and internal resource allocation within the hospital. His stance on these issues stemmed from emphasising that the overriding feature that makes hospitals different is that they are effectively *two* firms within one organisation. Although it had been recognised before that there was more than one line of authority in hospitals, Harris sought to analyse the nature of, the interrelation between what can be termed the 'doctor-firm' and 'administrator-firm' within the hospital. Essentially the patient care process is envisaged as a sequence of spot demands and delivery. On the demand side various doctors in the doctor-firm decide when patients need ancillary services, for example pharmacy, operating rooms, blood bank, etc., whereas on the supply side certain functionally orientated departments, for example pharmacy, stand ready to combine the necessary materials to produce and deliver the 'demanded' input into the patient care process. In effect, the supply function in the hospital situation is too specialised for the doctor-firm to handle alone hence the activities of the administrator-firm in ancillary service supply.

What distinguishes this process from the mechanic-firm role and the stores-firm role in the large garage or machine maintenance organisation? Harris argued that the hospital was unique because in the garage-type analogy the mechanic-firm and the stores-firm are 'on the same side', whereas in the hospital the doctor-firm must remain independent of the administrator-firm. The former's essential function is to provide the services that are *scientifically indicated* (emphasis in the original) and not to make repeated decisions about the costs and benefits to be expected at the margin from a particular unit of blood, therapy or test. The doctor must have, or appear to have, complete clinical freedom and therefore not be tainted by the resource-limited, business-orientated administrator-firm. This helps explain why hospitals are 'split down the middle'. In short,

> the doctor–hospital separation is intended to eliminate the necessity for repeated cost calculations in the clinical care of patients

> .... Hence, doctors get assured access to hospital inputs by becoming 'members' of the firm. Yet, unlike employees, they do not get told what to do. [Harris, 1977, p. 475]

Although the doctor-firm and the administrator-firm are really part of a single firm, there is a whole set of institutional constraints whose purpose is to 'make doctors look like individual entrepreneurs who happen to conduct their business on the hospital's premises' (Harris, 1977, p. 475).

If it is conceded that the hospital is two firms, the question is how are demanding and supplying roles co-ordinated, given that each firm will have its own objectives and constraints? Here Harris describes a world in which the solution to this problem is a non-co-operative oligopoly-type game. Two important consequences follow.

(a) The administrator-firm's short-run rationing of inputs involves a complicated system of uncodified rules, subtle manoeuvring, etc. In slack times this rationing process works satisfactorily; however, in more hectic periods of capacity and near-capacity demands the loose structure of rules-of-thumb contingency plans, side bargains, etc., tightens so that the administrator-firm effectively disciplines the doctor-firm's demand capacity by 'working to rule'; i.e., nurses do not provide therapies not in their contract, written requests are required for tests, the waiting list for in-patient care is adjusted, etc. In response the members of the doctor-firm seek to defend their share of available capacity by, for example, ordering a test in advance and cancelling it should it not be required.

(b) Harris, having noted the ability of doctors to demand inputs above the 'scientific minimum' that they regard as 'quality' improvements, pointed out that the doctor-firm and the administrator-firm will have different perspectives on the appropriate short-run capacity margins to meet uncertain demands. The administrator-firm will frown on unused capacity as a potential revenue loss and will want doctors to increase both cases and 'quality' (see Chapter 11 below for a discussion of the phenomenon in relation to health care cost inflation). The doctor-firm, on the other hand, is more content to keep a capacity margin for potential demands. These motivations set up pressures to expand the hospital size: the administrator wants a full hospital; but the doctors want bigger defensive capacity margins; the administrators will expand capacity only if it is to be filled; since there is an internal conflict over the defensive margins doctors within the doctor-firm will increase utilisation and 'quality' to maintain their shares; the administrators will hence allow the development of expanding empires within the doctor-firm and thus an expanding hospital. Harris derived some tentative policy conclusions from his model. A fairly obvious one is that hospital regulation policies directed at only one of the two firms will fail. Another, perhaps less obvious, is that doctors will use innovations to expand capacity and hence choose those innovations that expand the range of services that they can demand for their patients, rather than those that necessarily reduce resource use per case treated.

6.11 Summary

This chapter has focused on some of the reasons why economists have extended their approaches to the theory of the firm to give special attention to hospitals. The models discussed in detail, though only a small proportion of the wide range of approaches adopted, typify some of the major features of such models by their emphasis on the quality of hospital services and profit-making/non-profit behavioural differences. Apart from the Harris model, our discussion has implied throughout that there is a single decision-maker seeking a particular objective for the hospital. But in practice hospitals are highly complex organisations, comprising large numbers of separate decision-makers. Even in a centrally financed system such as the British National Health Service the principle of 'clinical freedom', the freedom of the doctor to take the course of action that he regards as best for his patient, leads to wide variations in the use of resources when we might expect greater consistency operating from the central government department. Each decision-maker, controlling a small 'province' of resources within the hospital, pursues his own objective, and the end result will be an inevitable compromise that emerges from the integration of separate decisions. Resources shared between different decision-makers will be allocated in a way reflecting the priorities and persuasiveness of each. With the possible exception of Harris, even the 'exchange' theories of hospital operation, which take explicit account of the interaction of different groups of decision-makers, have not produced a model of hospital activities that explains the multi-dimensional outputs of the modern hospital. Generally, what the theorists have achieved is the derivation of some implications about the role of quality in the modern hospital and the choice of methods and cases by different types of hospital. For a survey of many further implications of hospital models see Jacobs (1974). The effects of these implied outcomes on social welfare are not fully resolvable, but clearly they provide some justification for government intervention if individual preferences are overridden or equity pursued as a policy objective.

In the next chapter we consider the empirical evidence on hospital costs in order to derive some more practical implications about the 'industrial economics' of health care supply.

NOTES

1. The reader is asked to consider as an exercise which, if any, of the orthodox preconditions for perfect competition actually apply to the supply of medical care.
2. This is a familiar assumption in microeconomics which is introduced, as here, to ensure a 'sensible' market equilibrium. If the demand for care increased faster than the cost of providing it at higher and higher quality, then consumers would ultimately be prepared to buy an infinite amount of care of infinite quality (and price) – an implausible result!
3. One weakness of this result is its dependence on the elasticity of demand. If D_k is highly inelastic and D_l highly elastic, this result will not occur.

REFERENCES

CLARKSON, K. W. (1972) 'Some Implications of Property Rights in Hospital Management', *Journal of Law and Economics*, Vol. 15, No. 2 (October), pp. 363–76.

COCHRANE, A. L. (1972) *Effectiveness and Efficiency: Random Reflections on Health Services* (Rock Carling Fellowship Lecture). London: Oxford University Press for the Nuffield Provincial Hospitals Trust.

COOPER, M. H. (1975) *Rationing Health Care.* London: Croom Helm.

CULYER, A. J. and CULLIS, J. G. (1974) 'Private Patients in N.H.S. Hospitals: Waiting Lists and Subsidies', pp. 108–16 in Perlman, M. (ed.) *The Economics of Health and Medical Care.* London and Basingstoke: Macmillan Press for International Economic Association.

HARRIS, J. (1977) 'The Internal Organisation of Hospitals: Some Economic Implications', *The Bell Journal of Economics*, Vol. 8, No. 2 (Autumn), pp. 467–82.

ILLICH, I. (1976) *Limits to Medicine. Medical Nemesis: The Expropriation of Health.* London: Marion Boyars.

JACOBS, P. (1974) 'A Survey of Economic Models of Hospitals', *Inquiry*, Vol. 11, No. 2 (June), pp. 83–97.

LEE, M. L. (1971) 'A Conspicuous Production Theory of Hospital Behaviour', *Southern Economic Journal*, Vol. 38, No. 1 (July), pp. 48–58.

MATHER, H. G. *et al.* (1971) 'Acute Myocardial Infarction: Home and Hospital Treatment', *British Medical Journal* Vol. 3, No. 5770, (7 August), pp. 334–8.

MONOPOLIES COMMISSION (1973) *A Report on the Supply of Chlordiazepoxide and Diazepam.* London: HMSO.

NEWHOUSE, J. P. (1970) 'Towards a Theory of Non-profit Institutions: An Economic Model of a Hospital', *American Economic Review*, Vol. 60, No. 1 (March), pp. 64–74.

SCHWEITZER, S. and RAFFERTY, J. (1976) 'Variations in Hospital Product: A Comparison of Proprietary and Voluntary Hospitals', *Inquiry*, Vol. 13, No. 2 (June), pp. 158–66.

SKIPPER, J. K. JNR, SMITH, G., MULLIGAN, J. L. and GARG, M. L. (1976) 'Physicians' Knowledge of Cost: The Case of Diagnostic Tests, *Inquiry*, Vol. 30, No. 2 (June), pp. 194–8.

SPENCER, F. C. and EISEMAN, B. (1965) 'The Occasional Open-Heart Surgeon', *Circulation*, Vol. 31, No. 2 (February), pp. 161–2.

WILLIAMSON, O. E. (1963) 'Managerial Discretion and Business Behaviour', *American Economic Review*, Vol. 53, No. 5 (December), pp. 1032–57.

7 Estimating Hospital Costs

> What are the shapes of the short run and long run cost functions of hospitals? Are there economies of scale? The answer from the literature is clear: 'The exact general form of the function is unimportant' (Feldstein (1967) p. 133), but 'whatever its exact shape' (Ingbar and Taylor (1968) p. 107), and depending on the methodologies and definitions used, economies of scale exist, may exist, may not exist, or do not exist, but in any case, according to theory, they ought to exist.
>
> *S. E. Berki* (1972, p. 115)

7.1 Introduction

We have seen in the previous chapter how the quality of care provided has been a central theme in several economic models of hospital activity. It would be appropriate, therefore, in this chapter to examine the empirical evidence on the importance of quality for the costs of hospitals. This is not possible, however, owing to the major difficulties involved in attempts to assess the quality of care independent of other characteristics of hospital operation. These difficulties arise because the output of the hospital as a production unit is the improvement in the health of the patients treated. This output would reflect the quality of care in so far as it affected the patients' health (the obvious objective) but it is as yet unquantifiable. (For a discussion of approaches to the measurement of the output of health care, see Chapter 8 below.) Therefore, even where attempts have been made to adjust for quality, they are typically based on the quality of inputs to the patient and do not necessarily convey any information about the quality of the outcome.

This fundamental difficulty is sidestepped to an extent by concentration on inputs as the important elements in hospital behaviour and costs. The models presented earlier suggest that competing hospitals will attempt to increase the quality of care as perceived by patients in their hospital, for which purpose increasing the quality of inputs may be appropriate. But this does not resolve the problem for the cost analyst. Measuring input quality across a wide range of labour and technical inputs is not feasible and, if it can be done at all, can be done only by approximation. Thus, cost analysis suffers a major limitation by comparison with the earlier theory.

However, cost analysis has none the less been pursued on quite a large scale with a view to explaining the structure and rapid inflation of hospital costs (especially in the United States), albeit with limited use of quality as a dependent variable. Two particular problems have formed a focus for much of this activity in a *cross-section* context, i.e. the context in which the cost and 'output' of a large number of hospitals are observed for a particular time period. (The little used alternative process is to study the costs and 'output' of a given hospital over successive time periods. The latter is a *time-series* approach.) These are (a) the optimum size of a hospital, usually measured as the number of beds (i.e. testing for economies or dis-economies of scale) and (b) the relationship between average cost and marginal cost (this having implications for the optimum rate of utilisation of facilities). Analysis of these two issues is the focus of the discussion of empirical results later in this chapter. The analysis of empirical evidence on cost inflation, another area examined by econometricians, is deferred to Chapter 11.

However, before considering these aspects of the results, we will first revise the elementary cost theory involved and examine a number of methodological problems that affect the estimation of hospital costs.

7.2 The long-run average total cost curve and economies of scale

In elementary economic theory the shape of long-run average total cost curve (or planning curve) takes a U-shape, indicating the presence initially of economies of scale and later, at higher levels of output, dis-economies of scale. This possibility is illustrated in Figure 7.1. The section of the curve before *OQ**, the optimum size of the firm, indicates economies of scale; beyond *OQ** the curve rises, indicating dis-economies of scale. The most often cited source of economies of scale is the effect of a larger output enabling fixed costs to be reduced per unit of output.

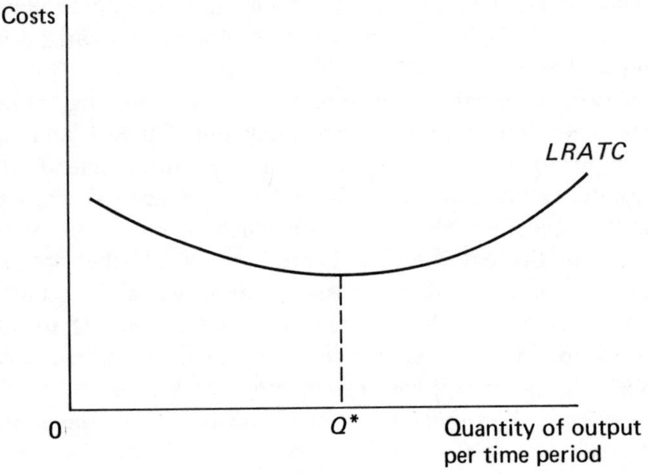

Figure 7.1 The textbook long-run average total cost curve

Other sources of scale economies are quantity discounts that may be negotiated on large purchases of inputs and a production function that for technical reasons exhibits increasing returns to scale. This will lower the average cost of factor inputs per unit of output for large quantities of output. Are there great possibilities for economies of scale in health care provision? As Fuchs (1974) points out, 'we need better estimates of how cost is related to scale of production before making definitive judgements about the advantages and disadvantages of encouraging group practice or other changes in organisation' (Fuchs, 1974, p. 148). He adds the important rider that, since the economic relationships change with the passage of time, they need periodic re-estimation once established.

7.3 The unit of output

Obviously, if we were examining the cost structure of any industry we would expect to find it stated in terms of the total cost, average cost or marginal cost of each quantity of output. Thus for the electricity supply industry, frequently analysed by econometricians, costs can be related to the kilowatt-hours of electric power produced. But we have already indicated above the difficulty of measuring the ultimate output of health services, the improvement in patient health, and so we consider here the alternative measures of what is sometimes termed 'intermediate' output used in estimating hospital cost structures.

Two appealing and widely used possibilities are the in-patient-day (or week) and the in-patient case. The first suggests that the hospital will increase its output with every extra day of patient stay; the second that it is the number of different patients treated that is the output that determines total cost. (In the UK cost per case and cost per week are widely used in hospital statistics. Feldstein (1967) points out, however, that their use interchangeably is not legitimate.)

Clearly, if the individual patient receives services daily that improve his health, then the patient-day is an appropriate proxy for the unit of output. The provision of meals and laundry, for example, contribute directly or indirectly to the welfare of the patient and will increase *pro rata* with length of stay. But while this measure fits the 'hotel' side of hospital services well, it takes no account of the likely time pattern of costs incurred by the hospital for the treatment of each case. Figure 7.2 shows a hypothetical cost profile for an individual case, showing costs incurred for each day of the patient's 'spell' in hospital. Areas designated *A* indicate the fixed costs of each case, such as the routine administrative and perhaps medical procedures of admission and discharge. *B* shows the hotel costs, for meals, laundry and the general staffing of the hospital, and *C* shows the treatment costs. These are hypothesised to rise to a peak relatively early in the patient's stay and then decline. Such a pattern is highly plausible for the simple surgical case, where surgery is followed by recuperation, initially with extensive supervision or intensive care but falling to only nominal supervision as the patient's health recovers. Obviously, the profile will differ for different types of illness. But even for

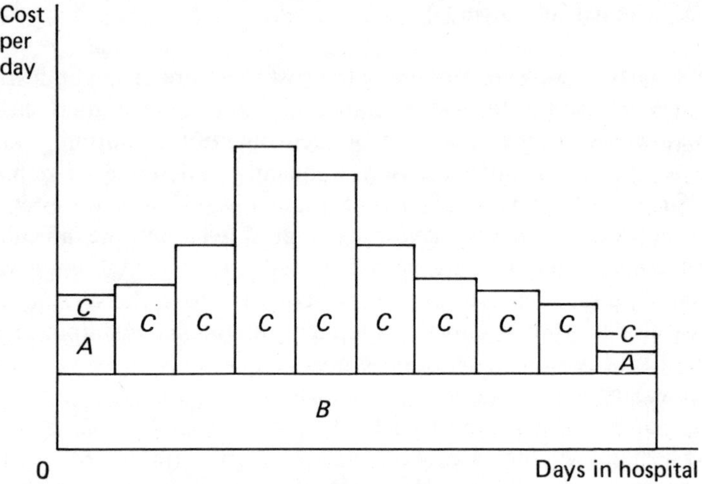

Figure 7.2 Hypothetical patient cost profile

cases that do not require surgery (unless they are long-stay cases, such as the mentally ill or the old), therapeutic activity is likely to reach a peak early in the treatment and to decline towards the end.

The implication of such a profile is that the patient-day is not wholly appropriate as a unit of output. An extra day of recuperation at the end of treatment is unlikely to have any substantial effect on the health of the patient and so its contribution to output will be small. Also, if the hotel costs are a small part of the total cost, as they may be where sophisticated treatment facilities are involved, the average cost per patient-day will not be the appropriate basis for a cross-section comparison of cost structure. The length of stay will affect the cost per unit in different hospitals even if the bulk of their costs, (i.e. for treatment) are the same.

In spite of these difficulties with the in-patient-day, we cannot unambiguously recommend the in-patient case as the unit of output. It has the advantage that any increase in the intensity of treatment that raises cost per day, while shortening length of stay proportionately more, is correctly reflected as an increase in efficiency by lowering cost per unit. But where it is not possible to detail the types of cases being treated, as is typical for many US studies, differences in case mix will alter cost per case in a way that cannot be explained by the cost equations. That is, if cost per case cannot be standardised for the types of cases involved, we will be estimating a cost structure across 'firms' that are not 'producing' a common 'output'. However, if the more difficult cases also have a longer stay in hospital (as seems plausible in general) owing to variations in the sophistication of treatment and the time required to recuperate, then the patient-day as a unit of output is crudely standardised for case type differences. That is, cost per day is cost per case adjusted for length of stay. Of course, if the simple linear relation between cost and lengths of stay does not always hold, as our previous discussion of the time profile of costs suggested, then cost per day will be an incorrect measure of cost per unit, biasing downwards the cost per unit of inefficient hospitals that retain patients for a longer stay than is clinically required.

The choice of units of output has been resolved in the literature pragmatically rather than by detailed theoretical analysis of each measure of output. Analysts able to standardise for the type of case treated (e.g. Feldstein, 1967; Evans and Walker, 1972) place greater emphasis on cost per case as a dependent variable, while others, predominantly working with US data (e.g. Lave and Lave, 1970; Ingbar and Taylor, 1968), use cost per week. Since it is the results on optimum size and utilisation that concern us here, we will not pursue the discussions of the unit of output further. However, it is worth noting that the analysis of cost per case with some account taken of differences in the types of cases treated is likely to explain more of the variation in hospital costs than cost per week analysis, which lacks such case mix data. But since this is due at least partially to the greater detail of data, we cannot conclude that cost per case is proved by the analysis to be more appropriate.

7.4 The efficiency of hospital operation

A further difficulty facing the cost analyst is that hospitals will not necessarily be operating in the most efficient (i.e. cost-minimising) way. The earlier theory suggested that quality of care was of paramount importance to hospital and consumer behaviour, with the likely result that the price becomes an indicator of quality to the consumer (indicating a positively sloped demand curve over a range at least). Thus, cost competition by private hospitals may be bad for business if it reduces the price of care, the proxy for the quality of care in the eyes of the patient. Public hospitals and private hospitals receiving their revenue from third parties, predominantly the government and insurance companies, are also not necessarily operating at minimum cost, since they do not face the direct discipline of competition. As a result, any estimation of cost functions will reflect what Evans (1971) calls behavioural costs rather than minimum costs. This may be a rather fundamental drawback if there are significant differences between the two, leading to mis-estimation of the true cost structure. However, it is a problem that most analysts are aware of, and, in the absence of any detailed evidence on minimum costs, the focus on behavioural costs is again the pragmatic solution.

7.5 The regression model

A final problem that must be considered before we look at the specific issues of size and utilisation is the question of the regression model to be used. The analyst has to decide what independent variables to include in order to explain the cost variation between hospitals and to isolate the significant variables responsible for such variation. If it was simply a test of a well developed theoretical model then the model itself would dictate the variables to be included. But, as we have noted, there is a substantial gap between theory and econometric analysis in this field. Econometric models of hospital costs are seldom specific on the relevant variables *ex ante*. Therefore, the analyst has at his fingertips not a well defined and theoretically significant set of variables, but data on a wide range of variables each of which *might* affect cost per unit.

Selection from the set of variables available is frequently carried out via the regression equations themselves. Different permutations from the independent variable set are included in regression equations for cost per unit. Those equations yielding statistically significant results are then taken by the analyst as the focus for his discussion of the effects of each variable on unit cost.

Clearly, any element in the hospital that is closely linked to unit costs will, when measured and included in the regression equation, typically yield a significant coefficient and increase $\bar{R}^2$, the proportion of the variation in unit cost explained by the independent variables. But if the argument is reversed and these statistical results are taken to imply that it affects costs directly, then the analyst faces the possibility of error in that the real cause of higher costs may be some other variable, unmeasured and possibly unnoticed. As a result, too much emphasis is applied to the wrong element in the hospital. A facetious example might make this clear. Suppose we measured numbers of clean white coats and rubber gloves used by a hospital and regressed average cost per case or per week on these variables alone, obtaining significant coefficients. Since the variables we have measured are related to staff, numbers of operations, etc., the coefficients showing the effects of an additional coat or pair of gloves on average cost would greatly overstate the direct cost of these items alone since the model would attribute the whole cost effect of additional operations to the rubber glove variable. Failure to include staff variables directly would therefore over-emphasise these particular variables.

We are not suggesting that such simple errors occur in the literature on the analysis of hospital unit costs. Indeed, the econometricians involved frequently go to some lengths to avoid them. The point is simply that, when the important cost influences are being identified not by theory but by results, every step should be taken to ensure that the relevant variables are being measured directly and are not concealed behind some other variable.

A further point worth noting, raised *inter alia* by Sorkin (1975), is that the studies are limited to a consideration of the costs incurred by hospitals, and therefore ignore costs incurred by staff, patients and visitors. Perhaps the most obvious example of costs incurred by staff, patients and visitors are travelling costs. Given that, as the size of hospitals expand, we could expect their service areas and hence travel costs also to expand, it is reasonable to expect that the inclusion of such costs would reduce the optimum size of hospitals.

7.6 The optimum hospital size

We can now return to our discussion of the first area of interest for cost analysis in the health field, the question of the optimum size for a hospital. The simplest econometric approach to this question involves relating cost per unit to a number of independent variables selected by the analysts as likely to be important influences on unit costs. Thus, where size is the main interest, an equation of the following form is the simplest beginning:

$$AC_i = \alpha_0 + \alpha_1 S_i + u_i \tag{7.1}$$

where AC_i = average cost per unit of ith hospital;
α_0 = constant to be estimated;
α_1 = coefficient to be estimated;
S_i = size of ith hospital;
u_i = error term.

The measurement of size itself poses methodological problems which we will not pursue in detail here. A number of authors use the number of beds available as a measure of capacity, but this ignores the role of staff and technical facilities, each of which could limit the effective capacity of the hospital. An alternative is to use the average number of patients per day in the hospital. This implies that the hospital uses its capacity to the limits imposed by one or more of the inputs, other than beds. This presumably implies that above-average patient numbers can be dealt with only if capacity is extended in some way, e.g. by staff working overtime. Since this would generate additional costs, the average level of activity is a more appropriate measure than the maximum number of patients.

Equation (7.1) implies that cost per unit will either increase or decrease with size and that minimum cost would be achieved at a size of zero or infinity! However, it is possible to parallel the usual assumptions for cost curves, i.e. U-shaped long-run average cost, within the linear regression equation by adding an additional term, giving

$$AC_i = \alpha_0 + \alpha_1 S_i + \alpha_2 S_i^2 + u_i. \tag{7.2}$$

The term in size squared (S_i^2), together with that in size (S_i), permits U-shaped cost curves to be estimated by ordinary least squares regression. This can be readily seen if we differentiate (7.2) to give

$$\frac{dAC_i}{dS_i} = \alpha_1 + \alpha_2 S_i .$$

For a familiar U-shaped average cost curve, the slope (i.e. the first derivative) will start off negative when size is zero, become zero at the optimum size and rise thereafter. Therefore, if

$$\frac{dAC_i}{dS_i} < 0 \; (S_i = 0)$$

and

$$\frac{dAC_i}{dS_i} > 0 \; (S_i \to \infty)$$

then it follows that

$$\alpha_1 < 0$$
$$\alpha_2 > 0$$

and, at minimum average cost,

$$\alpha_1 + \alpha_2 S_i = 0$$
$$\therefore \quad S_i = -\alpha_1/\alpha_2 .$$

Thus, minimum average cost will occur at a higher size, the greater the magnitude of $(-\alpha_1)$ relative to (α_2).

To confirm that this is indeed a minimum, the second-order condition gives

$$\frac{d^2 AC_i}{dS_i^2} = \alpha_2$$

which, since $\alpha_2 > 0$, confirms a minimum. If $\alpha_2 < 0$ and $\alpha_1 > 0$, then

$$\frac{dAC_i}{dS_i} > 0 \; (S_i = 0)$$

$$\frac{dAC_i}{dS_i} < 0 \; (S_i \to \infty)$$

and we have an inverted U- or bell-shaped cost curve, with average cost rising to a maximum and then falling. (This is confirmed by the second-order condition, $d^2AC_i/dS_i^2 = \alpha_2 < 0$.)

Finally, if α_1 and α_2 have the same sign then the slope never changes sign and average cost either rises (α_1, $\alpha_2 > 0$) or falls (α_1, $\alpha_2 < 0$) continuously with increasing size.

In practice, econometricians examining the question of size do not limit their analysis to an equation as simple as (7.2) above. To omit other relevant influences on cost may lead to a mis-estimation of the effects of size alone. Thus equations are normally built up to include a wider set of independent variables, of which utilisation is one.

7.7 Utilisation

The importance of the utilisation rates for hospital costs reflects the relationship between average cost and marginal cost. If the total cost of a hospital is largely made up of fixed costs due to, e.g., building, maintenance, minimum staffing levels, then cost per unit could be reduced if the facilities could be used more intensively. For example, if total cost for a given hospital was related to utilisation by a simple linear function

$$TC = K + MQ \tag{7.3}$$

where TC = total cost;
K = fixed capital/maintenance cost;
Q = number of patients (or patient weeks);
M = marginal cost per patient

then average cost per unit of output is

$$\frac{TC}{Q} = AC = \frac{K}{Q} + M$$

$$\therefore \frac{dAC}{dQ} = \frac{-K}{Q^2} < 0$$

which implies that average cost falls as the hospital is used more intensively.

In practice, a hospital is most unlikely ever to achieve a level of utilisation of 100 per cent of the available capacity. The treatment of patients in hospital is obviously subject to a great deal of uncertainty as to the date of admission and discharge of any given patient. Thus, if a patient makes a good recovery and is discharged earlier than expected, another case may not be booked to occupy the bed until a few days later and so it remains unused for the intervening time.[1] But utilisation approaching 100 per cent is worth striving for if fixed costs dominate variable costs in the total cost function.

Data on utilisation can be drawn from three closely related variables, occupancy, throughput and length of stay. Occupancy rates show the average fraction of the available capacity occupied per day; throughput rates show the number of patients treated per unit of capacity in one year; length of stay is obviously the average number of days spent by each patient in hospital. The three are related in the following way:

$$LOS = \frac{OCC}{THPT} \times 365 \qquad (7.4)$$

where LOS = length of stay;
OCC = occupancy rate;
$THPT$ = throughput.

Thus, length of stay falls if throughput increases for given occupancy and rises if occupancy increases with no change in throughput. (In other words, when a hospital uses given facilities more intensively then it must be discharging patients earlier, and when it uses more facilities for the same throughput of patients it must be keeping patients in hospital longer.) Given the close relation between these three variables it is tempting to select one as the best measure of utilisation. But each measures a separate dimension. Essentially we are dealing not with one marginal cost, as suggested earlier, but with two. We are interested in the cost of treating an additional patient. But this can be done in two ways, either by shortening the length of stay of patients or by increasing the occupancy of the hospital's capacity. Both can legitimately be termed changes in utilisation, the first of existing beds in use, the second of total capacity. These two ways of achieving the same end result may have different cost consequences, and so both need to be taken into account. However, length of stay will be affected by the mix of different case types treated by the hospital and so may not be included by some analysts, particularly when case mix has already been included separately in the regression equation.

7.8 Size and utilisation – empirical results

Rather than catalogue in full the results of the considerable number of econometric studies that have been carried out largely in America (see Berki (1972) for a full bibliography, and Sorkin (1975) for a concise summary), we will confine attention here to a few illustrative examples selected from Britain and America.

Feldstein (1967) produced the first major econometric study of English hospital services and his remains the dominant work in a subject that few have followed up in Britain. Feldstein had access to data not only on hospital costs and cases treated but also on local government health service provision. Thus, in the later chapters of his book he examined detailed multi-equation models of the whole system. He also fitted production function models to the data and examined an input – output approach, all with results that are of interest. But our focus here is the regression results obtained for size and utilisation.

Feldstein used data from 177 acute non-teaching hospitals, i.e. hospitals treating general short-stay medical and surgical cases, in England and Wales for the cost year 1960–61. For the regression analysis, size was measured by the number of beds available in the hospital rather than the total 'output' of patient days or cases. This has the disadvantage that it takes no account of the other factors, discussed earlier, that may effectively determine hospital capacity. In addition, Feldstein formed case-mix variables by calculating the proportion of hospital cases in each of nine aggregate categories.

Regression of average cost per case on the case-mix variables with size and size squared suggested a shallow U-shaped average cost curve with minimum average cost at 310 beds. But the interaction between different variables is particularly well illustrated by this result. Size (and case mix) as the only independent variables in the equation lead to a result suggesting that economies of scale are not particularly important (i.e., the average cost curve is shallow). But Feldstein investigated the relationship between size and utilisation and found that larger hospitals tended to have lower rates of utilisation (measured by throughput per bed). Extension of the regression model to

$$AC_i = \alpha_0\ BEDS_i + \alpha_1\ BEDS_i^2 + \alpha_2\ THPT + \alpha_3\ THPT^2 + \hat{\gamma} R_i \tag{7.5}$$

where R_i = vector of case-mix proportions and
$\hat{\gamma}$ = vector of estimated coefficients for each case-mix variable,

showed that the apparent absence of significant economies of scale comprised two effects. Increases in size and in throughput yielded lower average costs. Thus, for the larger hospitals, economies of scale were offset by the higher costs associated with their lower rates of throughput. In fact the results for economies of scale suggested that hospitals up to 900 beds would enjoy declining costs (12 per cent less at 900 beds than for the average of the sample) as long as they maintained throughput rates at the levels of smaller counterparts.[2] Increasing utilisation up to a rate of approximately thirty-two cases per bed per year would also reduce cost per case, according to Feldstein's results; i.e., marginal cost is less than average cost. Since Feldstein's data did not include capital costs and depreciation but only running costs such as heating and maintenance, we cannot automatically link this result to the fixed costs of providing hospital facilities initially. Instead we might link it implicitly, rather than through any demonstrable effects, to such things as staffing levels. These are typically linked to the number of beds and so most cases can be treated if staff members work more intensively.

By comparison with Feldstein's domination of a very sparse literature on UK hospital costs, no single US study suggests itself immediately as representative of the large body of work conducted on American hospital costs. Therefore we review two such studies as examples of other approaches. (For a broader review, see Berki, 1972).

Ingbar and Taylor (1968) adopted a more complex statistical

technique for their examination of hospital costs in Massachusetts to address the same questions concerning size and utilisation. Using principal components analysis they reduced their data, on over 100 different variables for seventy-two hospitals, down to fourteen key factors. Eleven of these were then related to the original variables by identifying those that were most highly correlated with factors. Size – volume, utilisation and length of stay are the three that interest us here, the remaining ones reflecting aspects of case mix or support services such as laboratory activity. In their regressions of cost per patient-day on subsets of these eleven variables, they obtained a theoretically perverse result. This was that maximum cost per patient-day was predicted to occur at a size of 150 beds. However, the difference in cost between this size hospital and the average was sufficiently small for a conclusion that average cost per patient day was virtually constant across hospitals of different sizes to be proposed.

For utilisation, Ingbar and Taylor used occupancy rates as their measure. As we have seen earlier, this is related to throughput via the length of patient-stay in hospital. But, while throughput shows variations in the intensity of use of the hospital, whether through using more beds or a shorter stay to accommodate a higher total number of patients, occupancy rates measure the use made of the bed stock only. Thus, a shorter stay and higher throughput of patients for a constant number of occupied beds would not be recorded by this variable as an increase in utilisation. The regression result, which showed that cost per patient day would be lower when occupancy rates were higher, is not particularly surprising, nor does it necessarily tell us a great deal about the relevant average and marginal costs. For if the higher occupancy is achieved by lengthening the patients' stay in hospital, a lower average cost *per day* (not per case) is predicted by the pattern of costs against time suggested earlier (Figure 7.2); i.e., the marginal cost of an extra day in hospital is less than the average cost. This has no particular implications for efficiency and utilisation, since if extra days in hospital may make no difference to health then their provision is inefficient. Alternatively, if more patients are being treated with constant length of stay, then greater utilisation of the hospital's capacity is contributing additional units of health care at a marginal cost below average cost.

Essentially, the confusion over the precise implications of the result arises because the units of output to which the costs refer are not clearly specified. Extra days of stay are not comparable with additional patients as units of output. Thus, throughput focuses on the latter while occupancy does not distinguish between them. Since we are more likely to be interested in the cost of treating extra patients, Ingbar and Taylor's result is not of itself convincing evidence on the marginal cost of providing this increase in output for their sample hospitals.

To sum up, Ingbar and Taylor's results for size and utilisation suggest that size is relatively unimportant and that higher occupancy rates will lower cost per patient day. While the first result may be accepted (though see Mann and Yett (1968) for a detailed criticism of their estimates of scale effects), the second does not shed a great deal of light because of the difficulty of interpreting it in terms of more intensive use of facilities.

A more recent study of US hospital costs by Lave, Lave and Silverman (1972) provided further evidence on the cost effects of size and utilisation through a highly detailed analysis of data on sixty-five hospitals. They began by specifying five elements that are likely to influence costs: (1) number of cases treated; (2) case difficulty; (3) quality of care; (4) hospital institutional characteristics; (5) capacity utilisation. The data available were classified into two categories, Characteristic and Diagnostic Variables. The 'characteristic' set included size, occupancy, teaching status and commonality of diagnoses (i.e. the percentage of patients with the same diagnosis). Although quality is included in their checklist, it is measured only indirectly in their analysis through variables such as teaching status, which is assumed to contribute to the quality of care. The 'diagnostic' set covers seventeen groups of diseases. These are aggregates that, though not providing homogeneity within each category, go some way towards achieving it within the constraints on the number of variables to be included in the regression equation. Lave *et al.* use average cost per case as their focus for analysis, again because of the standardisation permitted when case-mix data are available.

The initial regression equation regressed cost per case on fifteen characteristic and seventeen diagnostic variables. This equation was very successful in explaining variations in cost per case ($R^2 = 0.953$), but only four of the diagnostic variables had significant coefficients. Therefore, the original seventeen were reduced to five by aggregation. Three techniques were considered: principal components, clustering with principal components and clustering on estimated marginal cost. Only the third technique will concern us here, as it was demonstrated to be the most successful in predicting average costs per case in the sample hospitals for other years.

The first regression equation provided coefficients of the effect on average cost per case of each type of case, the marginal cost of each diagnosis group. Thus, if different types of case have very similar marginal costs then their aggregation into a single group, with a single coefficient in the regression equation, will not distort the results significantly (as long as the series of values of each case type is statistically independent of the other case-type series).

Turning to the results from the revised regression using the smaller diagnostic set, these confirm some of the findings reported earlier. The size variable has a negative and statistically significant coefficient indicating declining average cost per case as hospital size increases. However, the coefficient was very small in relation to the average cost per case in the sample, which suggests that economies of scale are present in larger hospitals without being of any great importance. (A U-shaped curve relating average cost to size was examined by adding size squared to the equation, but the earlier result was unaffected and size squared rejected.) The coefficient of occupancy was negative, confirming Ingbar and Taylor's result. However, since length of stay is included separately in the regression equation by Lave *et al.*, we are considering here a change in occupancy with constant average length of stay. That is, we are effectively examining the effect of treating more patients by using more of the available beds. This is equivalent to an increase in throughput per available bed and the result is in line with Feldstein's. The resulting coefficient was also of a similar magnitude to Feldstein's estimate, indicating that the marginal cost of an additional case was approximately 68 per cent of average cost.

Length of stay had a positive coefficient which showed that the marginal cost of an extra patient-day in hospital was approximately 5 per cent of average cost. This apparently confirms Figure 7.2 again. But the change in length of stay is considered with occupancy held constant. Thus, the small increase in cost per case becomes surprising because an increase in length of stay from 9.33 (the sample mean) to 10.33 would imply a reduction in the number of cases by one-ninth if occupancy remains constant, and hence an increase in the share of fixed costs borne by each case. To resolve this complication, we would need to know how far the two variables are systematically related. For example, if hospitals with high occupancy rates tended to have a longer average patient-stay, then collinearity would affect the separability of the regression coefficients for length of stay and occupancy. Unfortunately, the data provided by the authors do not permit further investigation of this point here. But the reader should note the difficulties of interpreting the relevant marginal costs of hospitals activity.

The three studies discussed above are just a small sample of the available literature. But they demonstrate two propositions that are typical. The first is that economies of scale are not of major importance in determining hospital costs. (See Berki's (1972) humorous, if somewhat cynical, conclusion quoted above.) The second is that higher utilisation rates, the treatment of more patients with given facilities, would permit the treatment of the existing patient numbers with fewer hospital beds (obviously) and, more significantly, at a lower aggregate cost. (Of course, more subtle effects might prevent this, e.g. the effects on staff morale and wage claims of a higher work rate.)

7.9 Summary

A brief and highly selective examination of the wide literature on hospital costs cannot hope to emphasise all the significant findings of such work. But two conclusions of some importance for policy-makers emerge clearly from the limited discussion here. The first is that economies of scale are not of any major significance in Britain or the US hospital sector. The second is that greater utilisation of existing facilities will lower the aggregate cost of treating a given number of patients or increase the number that can be treated in the given supply of hospital beds.

Two reservations remain, however. The quality of care has

not been satisfactorily incorporated into any of the regression models (see Feldstein (1974) for an attempt to adjust for output quality by standardising for input quality.) As a result, such analyses may be focusing on small differences in cost owing to scale or utilisation by aggregating across highly heterogeneous units of output, owing to differences in the quality of care. Such quality problems remain the major drawback to cost analysis.

As regards the policy relevance of the conclusions on size and utilisation, the increasing specialisation of medicine means that some treatment units exist that cater for the needs of only a small proportion of the population. Thus, if these units are to be of a viable size, and also need to share the operating and support facilities of a general hospital, then the size of new hospitals will reflect the minimum population catchment area that is appropriate for the most specialised forms of medicine. Of course, this 'critical mass' argument on size may not always be important, but certainly it is likely to exert an influence on hospital planning by private or public decision-makers.

More fundamentally, however, the results of this chapter indicate the need for more sophisticated planning of hospital usage, e.g. by computer control of waiting lists, already in use, in order to ensure that society makes the best use of the very large amounts of capital tied up in hospital buildings.

NOTES

1. A number of studies show that, even where beds are occupied, the capacity of the hospital is not being used effectively because large numbers of patients are occupying beds for non-medical reasons; e.g., patients fit for discharge may wait several days, particularly over weekends, before they are examined and discharged by a doctor, or some doctors may have a different standard for discharge and keep patients in bed much longer than their colleagues elsewhere. See Morris *et al.* (1968).
2. Since only three hospitals in the sample exceeded 900 beds in size, Feldstein concludes that his resultant minimum average cost is an artefact of the regression equation, with its term in $BEDS^2$. Therefore, using other functional forms, he shows that the hypothesis that costs decline monotonically (but not linearly) with the increasing size fits the data as well as the U-shaped average cost curve hypothesis.

REFERENCES

BERKI, S. E. (1972) *Hospital Economics.* Lexington, Massachusetts: Lexington Books, D. C. Heath & Co.

EVANS, R. G. (1971) 'Behavioural Cost Functions for Hospitals', *Candian Journal of Economics*, Vol. 4, No. 2 (May), pp. 198–215.

EVANS, R. G. and WALKER, H. D. (1972) 'Information Theory and the Analysis of Hospital Cost Structure', *Canadian Journal of Economics*, Vol. 5, No. 3 (August), pp. 398–418.

FELDSTEIN, M. S. (1967) *Economic Analysis for Health Service Efficiency.* Amsterdam: North Holland; also (1968) Chicago: Markham.

FELDSTEIN, M. S. (1974) 'The Quality of Hospital Services: An Analysis of Geographic Variation and Intertemporal Change', pp. 402–19, in Perlman, M. (ed.), *The Economics of Health and Medical Care.* London and Basingstoke: Macmillan Press for International Economic Association.

FUCHS, V. R. (1974) *Who Shall Live? Health, Economics and Social Choice.* New York: Basic Books.

INGBAR, M. L. and TAYLOR, L. D. (1968) *Hospital Costs in Massachusetts*, Cambridge, Massachusetts: Harvard University Press.

LAVE, J. and LAVE, L. (1970) 'Hospital Cost Functions', *American Economic Review*, Vol. 60, No. 3 (June), pp. 379–95.

LAVE, J., LAVE, L. and SILVERMAN, L. P. (1972) 'Hospital Cost Estimation Controlling for Case Mix', *Applied Economics*, Vol. 4, No. 3 (September), pp. 165–80.

MANN, J. K. and YETT, D. E. (1968) 'The Analysis of Hospital Costs: a Review Article', *Journal of Business*, Vol. 41, pp. 191–202

MORRIS, D., WARD, A. W. M. and HANDYSIDE, A. J. (1968) 'Early Discharge after Hernia Repair', *Lancet*, Vol. 1, No. 7544 (30 March), pp. 681–5.

SORKIN, A. L. (1975) *Health Economics*, Lexington, Massachusetts: Lexington Books, D. C. Heath & Co.

PART IV

Making the Best Use of Health Care Resources

8 Health Care, Cost Benefit and Cost Effectiveness Techniques

> The heady atmosphere of grand designs has to be replaced by the mundane, but ultimately more fruitful, ground of systematically applied economics – cost–benefit, cost effectiveness and output budgeting to improve the efficiency of allocation within extant institutions, . .
>
> *A. J. Culyer* (1971, p. 209)

8.1 Introduction

We have already reminded the reader several times that in a competitive market the quantity of any good or service produced is extended to its efficient point where the value put on an additional unit of output as given by the demand curve is exactly offset by the cost of producing an additional unit, the marginal cost. Generally the pressures of excess demand or supply will ensure the achievement of this equality. However, for public health care provision (as well as for education, defence and other public sector 'products') this automatic adjustment to the efficient quantity does not occur because the service is not largely bought and sold on the open market. To make up for this lack of knowledge of the efficiency or otherwise of increasing the output of public sector 'products', various techniques have been developed, the main one being cost – benefit analysis (CBA). Klarman has aptly described cost – benefit analysis as aiming 'to do in the public sector what the better known supply and demand analysis does in the competitive private sector of the economy' (Klarman, 1974, p. 326).

The basic idea of CBA is a simple one. It sets out to discover whether the benefits of a particular project outweigh its real resource (opportunity) costs. Only those projects for which there is a surplus of benefits over costs are recommended. Operationalising this idea, however, leads to considerable methodological and practical problems. After summarising the theoretical aspects of CBA, this chapter discusses these practical problems and shows how cost – benefit analysis and a less sophisticated variant, cost-effectiveness analysis (CEA), have been applied in the health care field. CBA as introduced in this chapter is viewed entirely as an efficiency technique. Readers interested in exploring a broader view, including equity considerations, should consult, e.g., Weisbrod (1968); Williams (1978).

8.2 Measuring costs and benefits: the theory

> There are two essential characteristics of cost benefit analysis: breadth of scope and length of time horizon. The first objective is to include all costs and all benefits of a programme, no matter 'to whomsoever they accrue', over as long a period as is pertinent and practicable. [Klarman, 1974, p. 326–7]

This section is concerned with the first problem, measuring all the costs and all the benefits. In economics the concept that deals with losses or gains of individual welfare as a consequence of a change in an economic variable is that of *consumer's surplus.* This can be defined as the difference between what the consumer would have been willing to pay for the units (of health care) he purchased and the sum that he had to pay. That is, when a consumption opportunity is provided to a consumer its value to him is the amount he would be willing to pay for it, which may exceed its market price. Similarly, when a consumption opportunity is taken away, for example to provide resources for producing some other good, the cost of this withdrawal is the amount the consumer would have been willing to pay for the consumption forgone. The concept of consumers' surplus has had a long and at times controversial history. Here we pay attention to a brief discussion of its role as a theoretical base for cost – benefit analysis. (For a fuller discussion see Currie, Murphy and Schmitz, 1971.)

Although consumer's surplus has been associated with a large number of possible measures – as many as twenty-seven according to Kamerschen and Valentine (1977) – we concentrate here on the compensating variation (CV) measure. Following Mishan (1975) we can state formally the basic principle of CBA. If a project makes someone better off, the appropriate measure of his benefit is his CV, the *maximum* he will pay rather than forgo the project. On the other hand if he is made worse off, his compensating variation measures the extent of his loss, being the *minimum* sum he will accept in order to put up with the project.

Theoretically, the compensating variation is measured by the area under the consumer's demand curve. This shows the amount he would pay for a given quantity of a good on a take-it-or-leave-it basis. Formally, we are dealing with a real-income constant demand curve when we measure consumer surplus rather than one for which money income is constant. This is because the project is either implemented or not and the gainers and losers get a fixed quantity, or nothing, of the good. A money-income constant demand curve, which could be estimated by observing the effects of a change in the price of the commodity, is affected by changes in real income. Suppose the usual price of a good is £1 per unit. If it goes up in price, consumers are worse off. Thus, their demand curve will reflect

(a) substitution into other goods, and
(b) the income effect of the higher price.

Therefore, while we are crucially concerned that our CV measure leaves the consumers neither better nor worse off, the money-income constant demand curve is based on varying real income. It follows that to estimate the appropriate CV requires the adjustment of available demand data by various approximating techniques. In addition the cost – benefit analyst faces the further difficulty that demand information does not exist for the good in question because of its nature, e.g. public supply. Thus he has to find alternative methods of deriving the CV's of consumers e.g. by questionnaire.

Given these difficulties, if in response to a particular project we find that

$$\sum_{i=1}^{n} CV_i > 0$$

then we know that the gainers from the project will gain more than the losers will lose. This indicates that implementation of the project will bring about a *potential* Pareto improvement. That is, if appropriate compensation took place via a costless transfer, no one would lose as a result of the project. However, compensation does not necessarily take place when public projects are implemented. The sum of the CVs indicates the potential gain. Its distribution is another matter.

8.3 Measuring costs and benefits: the practice

At least three possible methods of obtaining compensating variations that are in line with the 'preferences of individuals' approach can be identified. First, one could simply try to elicit the information from individuals directly by asking them. The direct question approach has two major drawbacks. The interviewee clearly has an incentive to act 'strategically' by giving false answers that bias the outcome towards his particular preference about any proposed health project. The further drawback is that, for Britain at least, people are familiar with the NHS and 'free' health services so that questions about 'willingness to pay' would probably mean little to them. Despite these drawbacks, recent years have seen developments in this approach. Jones-Lee (1976), for example, has obtained data on how individuals value their own lives using a sophisticated questionnaire technique. This is discussed below in Chapter 9.

The second method relies on the argument that the behaviour of individuals reveals their preferences and looks for implicit valuations. There are some instances in health care in which individuals are able to trade off time, for example, against extra money costs as in the choice of transport to clinic appointments. Observations of the trade-offs can be used as a guide to the appropriate valuation of time savings in health care.

The third and most popular method also relies on market observation. Here the aim is to look to market prices for surrogate measures of benefits or costs of a particular activity which have a fixed or certain relationship to actual benefit. For example, a common strategy is to collect data on lost working time and to argue that, if this can be retrieved by the adoption of some health care project, then its value is the wage rate for those hours. Needless to say, where markets exist for the health care inputs or outputs under consideration the appropriate information is readily available. However, the data may need adjustment if the market price is not thought to be the correct price because of, say, the influence of monopoly power, government taxes and subsidies or any other form of market distortion. In this case an adjusted 'shadow' price is used.

8.4 Classifying costs and benefits in health care projects

Although it is convenient to follow the normal convention and write of costs and benefits as though they are different, as we do below, it must be remembered they are in fact just two faces of the same coin. As Steiner (1974, p. 319) has pointed out: 'Because opportunity costs always represent benefits of a forgone alternative, there is no theoretical distinction between benefits and costs.'[1]

Four categories of costs and benefit are summarised in Table 8.1. However, it must be noted that this is a classification that relies on only two of the main distinctions commonly made. (For a much more sophisticated classification see Musgrave and Musgrave, 1976, Chapter 7.) The distinctions made here are between direct and indirect costs or benefits and tangible and intangible costs or benefits. Table 8.1 outlines these distinctions, both of which are to some extent arbitrary. The difference between direct and indirect is not a hard and fast one and hinges on whether the effect under consideration is directly related to the health project objectives or is a subsidiary consequence. The tangible item can be readily valued within the existing structure of markets whereas the intangible item cannot. Illustrations of the classification can be found in Klarman's (1965) classic study of the benefits (which are, of course, averted costs) of a programme to eradicate syphilis. Category (1), the direct tangible category, would be represented by the saved future medical expenses of treatment of syphilis as a consequence of a successful eradication programme. Category (2) encompasses the three D's outlined above in Chapter 2, namely the tangible indirect benefits that are the production (working time) gains that result from a reduction in lost working hours deriving from diagnosis and treatment. In this instance an allowance is made for the reduction of gross earnings that resulted from the reduced mobility and employability consequent on the social stigma of having been treated for syphilis should it become common knowledge. Category (3) would represent the direct intangible benefits of syphilis eradication in the form of reduced pain and suffering. Category (4), the indirect intangible benefit (not pursued by Klarman), might be represented by the aesthetic beauty of a well planned treatment centre for syphilis, designed by a Le Corbusier (hopefully without too much glass).

Table 8.1 A Classification of Health Care Costs and Benefits

	Tangible	Intangible
Direct	(1) Costs and benefits that are closely related to the project objective and can be valued in the market	(2) Costs and benefits that are closely related to the project objective and are not valued in the market
Indirect	(2) Costs and benefits that are not closely related to the project objective and can be valued in the market	(4) Costs and benefits that are not closely related to the project objective and are not valued in the market

It is worth noting that, roughly speaking, categories (1) and (2) correspond to what we termed pecuniary investment benefits in Chapter 2 (i.e., these are monetary type 'pay-offs' to health care expenditure), whereas categories (3) and (4) represent the consumption benefits. This is only 'roughly speaking' the case because, as Dowie (1970) has pointed out, consumption benefits are not necessarily ignored by the market so that they need not always be intangible in the sense defined here. For example, an individual's willingness to pay for health care will reflect his evaluation of both the 'investment' gain in work time and the 'consumption' gain of reduced pain and greater enjoyment of life. Thus the intangible psychic benefits will be included in willingness to pay in a perfect market. Category (1), then, may well include some consumptions benefits.

Estimates of direct and indirect tangibles are sometimes used as a minimum estimate of the benefits to be attributed to a health programme and are often termed the 'economic benefits'. This procedure is disliked by most health economists because it is often a misleading procedure to estimate benefits in a minimum way (even if the intention is to show that, even on a minimum basis, the benefits are greater than costs), and also because it fosters the erroneous belief that economists can only understand or are prepared to value market costs and benefits. Although it is true that the latter are very much easier to quantify, there is no case for arbitrarily excluding intangibles however difficult they are to evaluate.

8.5 Discounting and the time pattern of costs and benefits

It is important to note that the resource costs of setting up and operating a particular health project and the benefits associated with such a use of resources seldom, if ever, occur in the same time period. This is a problem because benefits incurred in this time period are likely to be preferred by individuals or society as a whole to benefits of an equal magnitude that occur in any later time period. Similarly, individuals do not consider costs of equal magnitude that occur in different time periods as identical, costs that occur in the future being preferred to costs that occur now. An obvious example is that we all like prompt payment of loans but are tardy payers of debts. Benefits and costs are therefore not considered independent of the time period in which they occur. A technique is required to take account of the fact that costs are typically incurred now while benefits accrue in the future. This technique is known as *discounting*. Costs and benefits accruing in future periods are scaled down to take account of the preference for present consumption over future consumption. Thus, a cost or benefit of size K occuring in year n has a present value of $K/(1+i)^n$ where i is a discount rate. The selection of this discount rate is a matter beyond the scope of this chapter. If B_0, B_1, B_2, etc. and C_0, C_1, C_2 etc. represent the money value of the benefits and costs in each period of the project life n years, the project yields a positive net present value (NPV) if

$$\frac{B_0 - C_0}{(1+r)^0} + \frac{B_1 - C_1}{(1+r)^1} + \frac{B_2 - C_2}{(1+r)^2} \cdots \frac{B_n - C_n}{(1+r)^n} > 0$$

i.e.,

$$\sum_{t=0}^{n} \frac{B_t - C_t}{(1+r)^t} > 0.$$

Where this condition is met the project is worth undertaking. It represents a potential Pareto improvement in that the sum of the benefits would more than meet the costs of the project and if distributed appropriately would ensure that no one was worse off following the project's implementation.

8.6 A framework for CBA

A framework of the basic steps in (health care) CBA has been provided by Williams (1974). Its reproduction, in essence, here serves three purposes: (i) to bring together into a coherent whole the rather wide-ranging discussion above; (ii) to facilitate the distinction between CBA and CEA made below; (iii) to provide a measuring rod by which to evaluate the examples of CBA and CEA presented below. The essential condition for carrying out CBA according to Williams are as follows.

(a) It must be possible to separate out one service from another in a way that makes sense. The main concern here is to define any project so that it addresses the policy question that is under consideration. Furthermore, all projects should be of optimal size in the sense that increasing the size of project by £1 on the resource cost side generates additional benefits (or reduces other costs) of £1 also. If the projects evaluated are not defined to be of optimal size, then the results of CBA can be misleading for resource allocation. The above of course supposes that projects can readily be altered in size along a continuum, which may not be the case.

(b) There must be a possibility of choice. Given that CBA and CEA are techniques designed to improve decision-making, this would seem an obvious precondition. Every budding economist knows that scarcity forces choices and the health sector is not immune from this basic economic problem of desires or wants exceeding resources. Hence, choice would appear to be ever present.

There are at least five types of questions within the health care sector to which CBA and CEA can in principle be directed:

(i) questions concerning *what* treatment or treatments should be given, if any, for particular conditions;

(ii) questions concerning *when* treatment should be available, i.e. the timing of care (questions of preventive medicine are obviously relevant here);

(iii) questions concerning *where* treatment should be given, e.g., should the mentally ill be treated in institutions or 'in the community', or, on a less grand scale, should paediatric out-patient clinics be held centrally at a large hospital or locally in smaller hospitals near to individual health service users' homes;

(iv) questions concerning to *whom* treatment should be given; for example, given a certain number of kidney machines and an excess of individuals who could benefit from their life-extending services, which patients ought to be selected for treatment;

(v) questions of *how* some techniques should be produced: this question revolves round different possible combinations of inputs to produce any given technique or treatment.

(c) It must be possible to identify the outcomes associated with alternative services. This is a problem in the area of health care economics where the economist is most vulnerable and has to rely on the information of the medical expert, although, as Williams observed, it may be possible to generate useful conclusions by simply making different assumptions about health care outcomes.

(d) It must be possible to value outcomes established at (c). The major point the economist makes here is that, given the scarcity introduced at (b) above, valuation is not optional: it is inescapable. All health sector decisions imply judgements about the relative costs and benefits of different courses of actions even if they are obscured by medico-bureaucratic interaction somewhere in the health sector. Indeed, as pointed out above, and below (Chapter 9), some CBA studies have erroneously sought these implicit valuations as sources of society's evaluation of costs and benefits.

(e) It must be possible to measure the cost of providing each service. Here it is the often elusive opportunity costs that are sought.

(f) It must be possible to convert the costs and benefits into common units of value so that their relative magnitudes can be compared. Basically this means that costs and benefits will have to be measured in money terms.

8.7 Measuring output in health care

The most difficult steps in the above are steps (c) and (d), measuring and valuing the outcome or output associated with the provision of a given health care service. Recent years have seen considerable progress in defining the nature of the output of hospitals and valuing it. The main contributions have been Fanshel and Bush (1970), Culyer, Lavers and Williams (1971), Rosser and Watts (1972) and Wright (1974). The first three of these works have a great deal in common although all are independent contributions. The basic insight is that what needs to be measured is the difference between what would have been the time path of an individual's health status without any health care intervention and the time path with care. The Culyer, Lavers and Williams approach is set up as follows and will be used as indicative of the other contributions. There are three steps in the analysis:

(i) setting up descriptive categories concerned with a patient's state in terms of pain-free social functioning;

(ii) a relative evaluation process that converts the descriptive categories into index points;

(iii) an absolute valuation process that converts the index points into money values.

As regards (i) ill health is seen as being composed of two components – intensity and duration. The former is further subdivided into pain (*P*) and restriction of activity (*RA*). First, intensity is classified by locating a given condition in *P–RA* space. In Figure 8.1 the vertical axis *OP* measures (notionally) increasing degrees of painfulness in terms of distance from the origin. The horizontal axis *ORA* similarly records increases in the restriction generated by a condition. Points C_0, C_1, C_2 and C_3 represent the *P*, *RA* ratings for given conditions. (For example, C_3 might be a hairline fracture of the leg with a relatively low *P* scale reading and a medium *RA* scale reading.[2]) The placing of different conditions in the *P–RA* space is to be achieved by asking medical experts to carry out the scaling (independently), continuing until a consensus is reached.

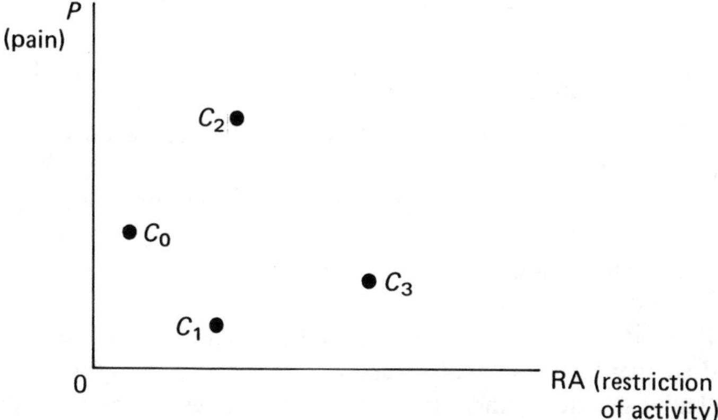

Figure 8.1 Classifying medical conditions by pain and restriction of activity

In order to convert the (*P*, *RA*) rating into a single intensity measure, combinations of *P* and *RA* that are equivalent in society's view (this may be proxied by medical opinion in practice) are assumed to be on an iso-intensity 'indifference' curve relating the two 'bads' *P* and *RA*. Figure 8.2 shows a set of such curves. Step (ii), the relative evaluation process, involves attaching a points scale to the iso-intensity curves. The suggested index of ill health involves a scale from 0 to 10 where

0 = normal;

1 = able to carry out normal activities, but with some pain or discomfort;

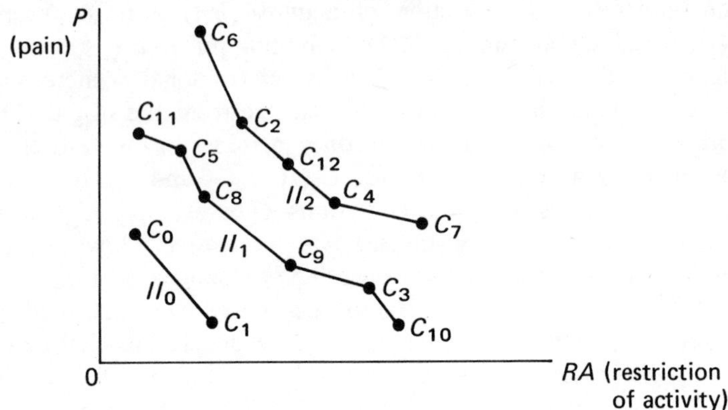

Figure 8.2 Developing iso-intensity curves

2 = restricted to light activities only, but with little pain or discomfort;
3–7 = various intermediate categories reflecting various degrees of pain and/or restriction of activity;
8 = conscious, but in great pain and activity severely restricted;
9 = unconscious;
10 = dead.

The index points are to be viewed as weights, not just ranks, and so they give cardinal measures of intensity. State 4 is twice as bad as state 2 and state 9 is three times as bad as state 3. II_0 II_1 and II_2 in Figure 8.2 above might then have weights 1, 2 and 3 attached to them. Once the index has been formulated and attached to the intensity categories, statistical estimates are then made about the time path (i.e. duration) of the intensity level with and without treatment, the difference being the output measure.

In the example illustrated in Figure 8.3, diagnosis takes place at time 0 and the first two post-diagnosis weeks are devoted to investigations and arranging treatment. In the absence of treatment the initial intensity index (5) rises sharply from week 7 to death index (10) in week 12. The time path of intensity with treatment compared to that without treatment is one of *increased* intensity from week 2 to 6 reaching a peak at intensity level 9 in the early part of the third week (this is the immediate adverse

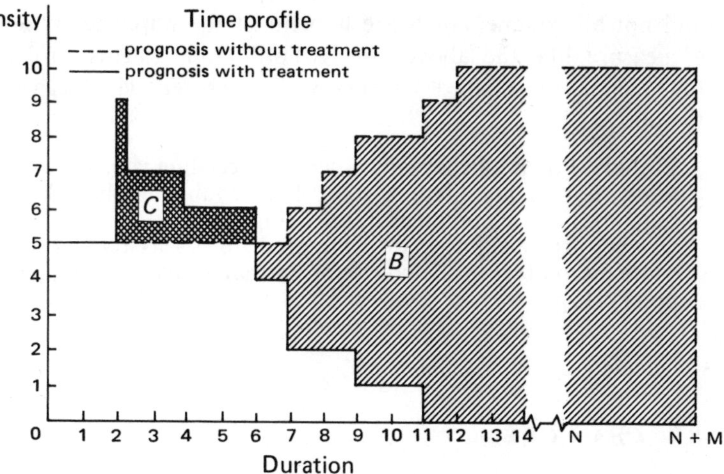

Figure 8.3 Measuring the output of health care

effects of an operation or other forms of treatment working themselves out). From week 6 onwards the intensity index continues to fall until index level 0 (normal) is happily re-established in week 11, and continues until death at the end of normal life expectancy at $N+M$ years.

The index score representing the effectiveness of this treatment involves subtracting area *C* (where intensity was worsened by treatment for a short period) from area *B* (where intensity was improved by treatment for a considerable duration). As a sophistication it is suggested that a present value of this output might be achieved by discounting:

> The primary purpose of such an indicator is to facilitate cost effectiveness studies, by providing a quantification of the purely humanitarian benefits to be used in conjunction with economic costs (and benefits) in order to improve the effectiveness of health services in the face of severe resource limitations. [Williams, 1974, p. 371]

The final step is to attach the money values to the index scores. The source of the money values is a difficult problem. Using implicit valuations derived from existing resource allocation, court awards or an arbitrary policy decision as a price per health 'point' are suggested as possibilities.

Output measurement in health care is still a daunting task,

and not all commentators are hopeful of the implementation of a measure like the above. Sir Richard Doll, Regius Professor of Medicine at Oxford University, has written with regard to the above:

> Frankly, I do not believe that such a proceeding is possible – certainly not in my lifetime .... The trouble is that different outcomes are incommensurate. Being dead is not, and never will be, just ten times – or a hundred times – as bad as having some discomfort in the course of normal activity. [Doll, 1974, pp. 11–12]

8.8 CBA v CEA

Enough has been said above to see that valuing and defining the output of health care provision is an extremely difficult task. It is not surprising that economists have looked to avoid some of the difficulties. One modification is to avoid Williams's step (d), the valuation process, by in effect holding the output or benefit constant, i.e. simply defining it in physical terms and looking for the least-cost way of achieving it. This is cost effectiveness analysis (CEA). The most celebrated example in the UK is probably that of Piachaud and Weddell (1972), who looked for the least-cost way of treating varicose veins. The output, varicose veins treated, was held constant and the least-cost method of treatment established.

At first sight this may seem to be a powerful technique, but there are some fairly severe restrictions associated with it. The major drawback is that the knowledge of whether the provision of a given health care technique is efficient or not is lost. The results of cost effectiveness studies simply give the least-cost way to achieve the desired end. They do not examine whether even in the least-cost method the costs actually outweigh the benefits. Therefore, they do not indicate whether it is at all worthwhile to provide the therapy that is under consideration.

A second major difficulty is that it is not easy to hold the output constant, so that, in the varicose veins case, for example, subsequent investigation suggested that the cost-effective method of treatment (injection compression sclerotherapy) did not have as long-lasting results as the cost-ineffective method (surgery) (see Hobbs, 1974). A further drawback to CEA is discussed in Section 8.8.1 below.

Although in Section 8.6 above five possible questions for CBA and CEA are outlined, it has recently become customary to classify studies under three headings (see Roberts, 1974; Williams, 1974; and Drummond, 1977). The more restricted classification distinguishes: alternative types of care, alternative places of care and alternative times of care. The distinctions are not mutually exclusive; for example, different types and places of care are likely to go together. However, they do provide a convenient classification.

Studies of alternative types of care include Piachaud and Weddell (1972), and Klarman, Francis and Rosenthal (1968), discussed below. CBA and CEA studies of alternative places of care are less common. Wager's (1972) study of care for the elderly is the most cited example. (A summary of Wager can be found in Williams and Anderson, 1975.) Alternative times of care bring preventive medicine to the fore. A distinction is usually drawn between primary and secondary prevention. The former is concerned to prevent or lower the risk of illness occurring as with vaccinations. The latter concentrates on the early detection and treatment of ill health. Screening procedures like mass miniature radiography fit into this second subcategory. Examples of alternative times of care involving primary prevention are Pole (1971) on the detection of tuberculosis and Robinson (1971) on the prevention of rheumatic fever.

Below two case studies are presented to give an indication of the practice of CEA and CBA in health care. The first case study concerns alternative types of care for treating chronic renal failure and is a CEA. The second is a recent UK study involving secondary prevention and is a CBA of a screening programme to prevent the birth of infants with Down's syndrome (mongolism).

8.8.1 Different types of care: treating chronic renal disease (CEA)

Klarman, Francis and Rosenthal (1968) addressed themselves to the question, 'Under existing conditions of knowledge regarding the cost and end results of treating patients with chronic renal disease, what is the best mix of centre dialysis, home dialysis and kidney transplantation?' (p. 4). It is a cost-effectiveness study, i.e. concerned with identifying the least-cost way of achieving a given (desirable) objective or objectives.

At the time of the study there were perhaps 6000 deaths per annum in the United States owing to chronic renal disease which could have been deferred through treatment. It was estimated that approximately 1000–1100 received available treatments – the overwhelming majority, 850, were on dialysis (the purification of the patient's blood by artificial kidneys) and 150–200 received transplants annually. The latter costs $13,000 per operation and the former $14,000 per annum at hospital (teaching or community) and $5000 per annum at home.

The main difference between the two distinct types of treatment is that dialysis continues over the patient's lifetime whereas transplantation, accepting that the follow-up period is long, is a 'one-off' treatment.

When transplantation is unsuccessful, the patient may revive and can have a further transplant operation or shift permanently to dialysis at home or in hospital. The (desirable) outcome or output of both procedures is life-years gained although, because with an effective transplant the life of the beneficiary is more 'normal' than with continuing (home or hospital) dialysis, life-years gained by the former procedure were weighted at 1.25 the life-years gained by dialysis.

The costs of the alternatives were measured in terms of the present value of lifetime expenditures for two cohorts of equal size (say 1000) each embarking on treatment with dialysis or transplantation. The costs depend on the expenditures given above and the volume and timing of services used. For the transplantation cohort life-years spent on dialysis subsequently by members of this cohort whose transplantation failed were considered. Drug costs were also included and future costs were discounted at a rate of 6 per cent.

The discount rate was adjusted to allow for the differential rate of unit cost increase anticipated. Because hospital dialysis and transplantation have a high labour component, they were attributed a 100 per cent higher rate of increase of unit costs at 2 per cent than for home dialysis. The net rates of discount became 5 per cent and 4 per cent respectively.

The major information requirement was survivorship tables giving years spent in dialysis and years with a functioning transplant. Experience of either type of treatment was too short at the time for life expectation to be anything more than speculative beyond the early years. The data source was an expert Committee on Chronic Kidney Disease (1967). Given assumptions about survival rates, the life expectancy gain for an individual entering the transplantation cohort was approximately 17.2 years – 13.3 additional years on a successfully transplanted kidney and 3.9 years on dialysis. For dialysis alone the life expectancy of the cohort was almost half at 9.0 years. This difference was accentuated when the 1.25 quality of life index was applied to the former figure. Table 8.2 summarises the calculations of cost and life-years gained for each cohort assuming a 50/50 split between home and centre dialysis for the dialysis cohort.

Table 8.2 Present Value of Expenditures and Life-Years Gained per Member of Cohort Embarking on Transplantation and on Centre and Home Dialysis

Modality	Present value of expenditures $	Life-years gained	Cost per life-year $
Dialysis			
Centre	104,000	9	11,600
Home	38,000	9	4200
Mean	71,000	9	7900
Transplantation*			
Unadjusted	44,500	17	2600
Adjusted for quality	44,500	20·5	2200

* The cost of transplantation incorporates $24,500 for dialysis, based on a 50-50 per cent distribution of patients between the centre and home

Source: Klarman *et al.* (1968)

It was apparent that transplantation was the more effective way to increase life expectancy of persons with chronic kidney disease at a given cost. A limitation on extending transplantation was a lack of kidneys and problems with storage, preservation and tissue-typing, constraints that might be eased by legal changes and improvements in medical technology. Improvements in dialysis would of course increase its relative attractiveness. With dialysis it was also clear (within the limitations of the available data) that encouraging home dialysis as opposed to hospital dialysis would be a resource-saving strategy. However, it must be noted that at the time of the study 100 per cent home dialysis was not practicable.

Comment. This study illustrates the strengths and weaknesses of CEA. The main strength is that a clear-cut and valuable result can be derived. The weaknesses are those that are common to the technique of CEA. (a) Adjustment had to be made to equate the 'output' of the dialysis and transplant techniques, the latter receiving a 25 per cent greater weight. This is clearly arbitrary but it must be noted, as the authors point out, that altering this 'weight' does not affect the rank of desirability of the alternatives. (b) No knowledge is gained on whether the benefits exceed costs of any of the forms of intervention to help patients suffering with chronic renal failure. Given the latter limitation, it is impossible to compare provision of transplantation facilities with any other desirable health or public sector project, as could be achieved with cost – benefit analyses on potential health and public sector projects.

8.8.2 Different times of care: preventing the birth of infants with Down's Syndrome (CBA)

In a detailed recent study, Hagard and Carter (1976) undertook a cost – benefit analysis of preventing the birth of infants with Down's Syndrome. Their stated aim was to estimate the costs and economic benefits of providing routine prenatal diagnosis of Down's Syndrome with termination of affected pregnancies in older pregnant women, in the west of Scotland. The method used involved five states:

(i) estimates of the number of births affected by Down's Syndrome by five-year maternal age groups in the area;
(ii) estimation of survival rates and degree of handicap;
(iii) estimation of costs to society of caring for survivors;
(iv) identification of the characteristics, including the number of affected births prevented, of a prenatal diagnosis programme;
(v) estimation of the costs of running such a programme.

(i) to (iii) are expected costs to be incurred by society by the birth of children with Down's Syndrome. (iii) and (iv) determine the expected resource saving from preventing affected births; the latter were estimated for 'replacement' (in which termination is followed by a further pregnancy assumed to be normal) and the 'non-replacement' case (in which women do not become pregnant again after termination). All costs were standardised to a value for July 1974 and a 10 per cent discount rate (currently used by the UK Treasury) was used.

Using a high rate of expected incidence of Down's Syndrome over the twenty-year range of maternal age, it was estimated that 5.4 per cent of all births, but 29 per cent of births with Down's Syndrome, would be to women aged thirty-five and over and 1.1 per cent of all births but 16 per cent of births with Down's Syndrome would be to women aged forty and over.

The benefits of a prenatal programme were interpreted as the averted costs. '*The economic benefit of preventing the birth of handicapped people is the cost to the community of their care.* In the case of abortion followed by a successful normal pregnancy (replacement) this is the difference between the cost of caring for a handicapped person and that of caring for an average person. When there is no further replacement the cost is the total cost of caring for a handicapped person (Hagard and Carter, 1976, p. 754 – our emphasis).

In estimating these costs the use of resources by a nominal cohort of 100 people live-born with Down's Syndrome was assessed. An estimate of the costs incurred is given in Table 8.3 for representative years for the replacement situation. They are made up under four heads by Hagard and Carter as follows:

(a) *Permanent care.* It was estimated that a quarter of patients would be in permanent care by the age of fifteen, half by the age of twenty-five, three-quarters by the age of thirty-five and all by the age of forty-five. The additional costs of permanent care over residence at home is higher for children than for adults partly owing to education costs.

(b) *Education.* In general, children with Down's Syndrome with IQs over 50 (20 per cent) attend special schools while the remainder attend occupational or day care centres. For those continuing to live at home special education was estimated to cost £100–£400 more per child per year than normal schooling,

Table 8.3 Costs of Caring for Cohort of 100 People Live-born with Down's Syndrome in the Replacement Situation

		Permanent care			Maternal income					
Age	No. of survivors	No. (%) in care	Cost (£)	Cost of education (£)	No. of children living at home	No. (%) of mothers unable to work	Cost (£)	Additional costs (£)	Total (£)	Present value (discounted at 10%) (£)
1	76	4 (5)	4588						4588	4171
2	73	4 (5)	4588		69	6 (9)	6660		11,248	9295
3	71	4 (5)	4588		67	6 (9)	6660		11,248	8451
4	69	3 (5)	3441		66	6 (9)	6660		10,101	6899
5	69	5 (7)	5735	23,560	64	12 (19)	13,320		42,615	26,460
10	65	8 (13)	9176	20,913	57	11 (19)	12,210	−4880	37,419	14,425
16	59	14 (23)	3528		44	12 (27)	13,320	43,939	60,787	13,227
20	55	13 (23)	3276		42	11 (27)	12,210	61,279	76,765	9514
45	27	27 (100)	6804					89,326	96,130	1317
									Total	£415,000

Source: Hagard and Carter (1976)

£10,000–£25,000 more a year for a birth cohort of 100 (replacement and non-replacement).

(c) *Lost maternal income*. It was assumed that the labour force participation among mothers of children with Down's Syndrome would be half that of average mothers with children of the same age. Using published wage and employment data it was estimated that six mothers out of 100 would forgo total potential earnings of over £6000 when their children were young, and eleven to fifteen mothers would forgo around £14,000 a year later on (replacement and non-replacement).

(d) *Additional costs*. Because of lack of data on the greater physical morbidity of those with Down's Syndrome the authors omitted these possible costs from the calculations. The inability of most people with Down's Syndrome to work, however, imposes a considerable economic burden on society. It was assumed that only those with IQs over 50 could work (i.e. about 25 per cent or less of those affected), and then with only half the productivity of the average person. Using average lifetime earnings and consumption data it was calculated that in the replacement situation for a birth cohort of 100 this would impose total costs rising from about £45,000 a year at age sixteen to a maximum of about £110,000 a year at age twenty-five.

Total averted costs (= *benefits*). Estimates of the total annual costs in each age group were obtained by adding the estimates under each heading for each year. In replacement situation and for a birth cohort of 100 they were calculated to increase from under £5000 a year in infancy to over £120,000 in middle life. The net present value for caring for a cohort of 100 people was £41,500 or £4150 per person in the replacement situation and £10,620 per person in the no replacement.

Costs of a prenatal diagnostic programme. The authors calculated the costs of a programme to examine 550 women *aged forty and over* each year covering the costs of work time lost, medical genetics provision, publicity, travelling and laboratory facilities. These women were estimated to be at risk of having 9.1 live-born infants with Down's Syndrome. Assuming 90 per cent would attend the clinic at the appropriate time for diagnosis, and with a diagnosis success rate of 99 per cent, the number of cases identified would be 8.1 (99 per cent of 90 per cent of 9.1). The estimated net present value of total costs of establishing and maintaining a twenty-year diagnostic programme was £311,855.

Comparing costs and benefits. The programme would prevent 8.1 children's births with Down's Syndrome and in the course of a Down's Syndrome programme one each year with myelocele.[3] In the replacement situation this would produce an annual economic benefit of

$$(8.1 \times £4150) + (1.0 \times £3940) = £37{,}555$$

and, over the twenty-year period, a discounted total of £351,699. For Down's Syndrome alone in the no-replacement situation the corresponding sum would be £805,587. Hence economic benefits would exceed the discounted costs of £311,855, supporting a test programme for pregnant women over forty.

Comment. This study is an attempt to do a CBA in what is obviously a sensitive and difficult area. In classifying the study as one of secondary prevention we are viewing the mongoloid foetus as an illness or rather a disability, to be 'treated' by the death of the foetus. Clearly, this approach to Down's Syndrome will be anathema to many people. However, the very least that can be said for Hagard and Carter is that they have opened up the issue for constructive discussion.

What are the limitations of the study? It will be clear from our earlier classification of costs and benefits that the authors have a very narrow conception of economic benefits, defining the latter as the direct and indirect tangible consequences of avoiding the birth of a mongoloid child. In doing so they have misrepresented the scope of CBA. (To do so in a medical journal compounds the error.) It appears that they have ignored many non-tangible benefits. A major direct intangible benefit of the prenatal programme would be a reduction of uncertainty. If you are over forty and pregnant, you and your family can be relieved of the uncertainty that you will or will not have to adjust your life-style to cope with a handicapped child. Some evidence that some consultant obstetricians think along these lines is provided in Forster (1977), from evidence of a survey of all consultant obstetricians in post on 1 October 1975 with the Trent Regional Health Authority.

> Rather surprisingly, one fifth of consultant obstetricians considered (8 out of 38) that it was not necessary to enquire before amniocentisis whether the patient would have no objection to an abortion if a severe abnormality was found. This suggests that these consultants viewed reassurance of the mother as the principal benefit of the test since there could be no guarantee that the mother would accept the offer of an abortion if an abnormality was detected. [Forster, 1977, p. 182]

There may well also be a gain from the relief of uncertainty (presumably) of a smaller magnitude at the individual level (but perhaps absolutely more important once aggregated over the relevant population) for all those women who run a risk of becoming pregnant in later life, and who would be screened should they actually become pregnant, an 'option' demand. There are also indirect intangibles to be considered. The birth of a mongoloid child is going to affect the parents' life-style in two ways. That their labour market contribution is likely to be inhibited seems clear, and the authors have rightly used a proxy for the lost market activity. But what of non-market adjustments? Households are themselves producers of goods and services including leisure. Production is achieved by combining market-purchased inputs with own time, and any interruption of this process is likely to have a value greater than zero. Furthermore, *if women have a choice* to work or not, then the observation that a proportion choose not to implies they rank the non-market alternatives as a greater source of utility. To look only to the working group for lost benefits is to underestimate.

Generally, it seems that the calculated B/C ratios are very much smaller than a fuller study would indicate. It cannot be argued that this is nit-picking, because in the study the B/C ratio for the over-thirty-fives in the replacement situation was less than 1, indicating the programme would be an inefficient use of resources. However, given the above, this result is tentative.

Formally, the study should have been concerned with what those individuals in the West of Scotland affected by the prenatal programme would be prepared to pay rather than forgo it. Clearly some of the data collected and analysed by Hagard and Carter are relevant, but they give the misleading impression that the scope of CBA is a narrow one.

Two complications with this sort of study loom large. First, what is the role of the foetus: is he part of society? Can we ignore his CV? Should we impute a CV for him? The answer to this appears to hinge on answering the question of when a small bundle of molecules becomes a human being and hence part of society, which is clearly an extremely difficult question, certainly beyond the scope of this discussion. (For a discussion of who is part of society see Dowie, 1970).

Second, what about those parents and friends of mongoloid children who write and give interviews to radio and television indicating that, although in the *ex ante* situation they would not have welcomed the child, once they had adjusted their life-style the child was able to have a meaningful and enjoyable life and that they had benefited greatly because the presence of the child had made them more loving, caring, less selfish and much more constructive human beings, etc? The status of this difficulty seems identical with that found in the economics of education, where it is agreed that education provides a desirable consumption good in the form of enhanced leisure in future periods. As Blaug (1970, pp. 20–1) observed, following Peacock and Wiseman (1968)

> It is perfectly true that there is an extraordinary consensus in most societies on the positive psychic benefits of education but, of course, it is a consensus of educated people whose taste for learning has been affected by the learning process itself. It is not so much that the belief that education makes for a richer life is a value judgement that lies outside the domain of empirical knowledge, but that it is *ex post facto* and hence of a different kind from the *ex ante* value judgement that governs the choice to acquire more education. [Blaug, 1970, pp. 20–1]

The thrust is that what matters in economic decision-making is the *ex ante* situation, and applying this to our present problem means that it is the *ex ante* CVs of *potential* parents of mongols that is relevant and not the *ex post* beliefs of parents and friends of mongol children. This however is perhaps too simple an appreciation of the issue, and some (see Section 9.5) would argue that to be a relevant technique CBA based on *ex ante* valuations must yield results that correspond closely to *ex post* valuations; i.e., can CBA be sensibly divorced from the *realised* consequences of a project?

8.9 Some criticisms and reservations of CBA and CEA

According to Meek, 'Cost – benefit analysis is a phenomenon, like Mr Enoch Powell,[4] which possesses a peculiar capacity to provoke wide differences of opinion about its utility' (Meek, 1972, p. 165). If this is true for cost – benefit analysis in general, one suspects the need to substitute two Mr Enoch Powells to parallel the controversy generated by the application of CBA to health care in particular.

8.9.1 Discounting

The rationale for discounting future benefits and costs, discussed above, is fundamentally that individuals prefer consumption now to consumption in the future financed by the forgoing of present consumption. (For a detailed discussion see, e.g., Dasgupta and Pearce, 1972.) The broadest justification is that anticipated increases in real income make the loss of utility from deferring present consumption greater than the gain from additional future consumption since future consumption is expected to be greater than present consumption for the population as a whole. There are of course additional justifications such as that consumption now is a certain prospect while consumption in the future is uncertain owing to the risk of death or failure of the investment. But we concentrate here on the rising real income argument and its importance for the evaluation of health care.

Growing affluence may make us less concerned about the cost of a hospital or treatment programme in the future. But what of its benefits? If these involve the saving of life or the avoidance of disability, it is by no means clear that these will be less highly valued because of greater affluence. Indeed, one of the characteristics of the very rich in the present time period is their tendency to spend very large sums of money on their health (see your newspaper's gossip column for a list of recent operations!). It is plausible to argue instead that health, along with other aspects of 'the good life', such as a pleasing environment, will be more highly valued in future. Depending on the growth rate of their value as income rises, a zero discount rate or even a negative rate might be appropriate. Therefore, the valuation of the future benefits of health care programmes and their discounting may not be as unambiguous as the benefits of investment programmes yielding more straightforward outputs such as electricity or water supply.

8.9.2 Criticism by non-economists

Some non-economists have been very disparaging about the technique of CBA. A selection of criticisms (see for example, Dror, 1967, and Self, 1970) have been answered by Williams (1972). However, as indicative of the non-economists' viewpoint, some issues raised by Draper and Smart (1974) are presented here. The authors consider the social sciences in relation to their contribution to the bureaucratisation of the National Health Service. As regards economics, Glass's (1973) review of CBA is taken as an example of the trend towards increased attention to cost – benefit studies and health economics research. Draper and Smart comment on Glass's article as follows: 'The approach advocated is perfectly in tune with the development of the techno bureaucratic control of health planning by obscuring the real problems in a hotchpotch of 19th century economic thought' (Draper and Smart, 1974, p. 459). The authors considered that CBA cannot cope when, as with health care, concern is with benefits to society as a whole. It is not so much that 'social benefits' are not easily measured but rather that 'there are virtually as many judgements as what to count as benefits to society as a whole as there are people in that society' (Draper and Smart, 1974, p. 459). Their point is that members of society may have very different and conflicting views such that the preferences of members of the community as regards the benefit of health care cannot be aggregated – health goals are plural. Glass's emphasis on the market as a source of information on values is attacked because the market economically exploits some, e.g. female health care staff, and fails to value others at all, e.g. pensioners. Further, it is argued that more emphasis should be placed on a comparison of health care expenditures and other public sector projects (e.g. Concorde).

Rather than CBA making clear the basis of any recommendations, Draper and Smart suggest that some would argue that 'such studies more often tend to mystify and obscure the nature of policy decisions and that the readily quantifiable factors tend to dominate the decision making' (Draper and Smart, 1974, p. 460). A broadening of discussion to include ecologic problems and social and political science is required, in their view, for CBA to be put in perspective.

Readers of the above sections should realise that most of the criticisms levelled at CBA are largely unfounded, although it is to be admitted that there are examples of studies that fall *far* short of an ideal CBA. But as Williams (1972) points out, the objective of CBA is to assist choice, *not* to make it, and although its limitations must always be emphasised the opportunity cost of not using it (in the form of more imperfect alternatives) is very high.

8.10 Summary

This chapter has attempted to cover a lot of material and, given the space limitations, has not done justice to the literature on many of the points raised. However, it is hoped that enough has been said to give the essence of the nature and use of CBA and CEA in health care.[5] It is worth noting that the last decade has seen, for Britain at least, a great increase in the size of the public sector, and hence CBA and CEA should become of increasing importance in the future. It is also worth noting that it has been argued that this increase in the public sector has not been paralleled by an increase in those public sector 'outputs' that are valued by society's members. This further strengthens the case for CBA in the whole of the public sector, not just the health care sector, in order to evaluate its performance comprehensively (see Bacon and Eltis, 1976).

Health care is an emotive area, and the studies reviewed in this chapter highlight some difficult moral issues concerning the valuation of such things as a prevented birth of a handicapped child and the extension of life for renal disease patients. Many find even the suggestion of such valuation highly unpleasant. But the economist's defence of CBA is like the comment sometimes attributed to Maurice Chevalier, who when asked how he viewed the prospect of old age replied: 'It's not exactly ideal, but it's better than the alternative.' (McKean, 1965). If decisions are not made in an explicit, if incomplete, way by CBA, then they will be made implicitly and may lack the kind of consistency necessary to obtain the best use from limited health care resources. A commitment to do everything possible for the dying is only a small commitment when little can be done. But the current environment of high technology and high-cost medicine makes such an absolute commitment, without regard to the relative benefits of alternative uses of resources, untenable in practice.

NOTES

1. Statements like 'Benefits are more difficult to measure than costs, . . .' (Ward, 1975, p. 111), are misleading. Steiner (1974, pp. 319, 320) argues that, 'it is not benefits that are difficult and costs that are easy to measure. Where market evaluations exist and are regarded as acceptable, measurement is easy whether on the benefit or cost side. Difficult cases occur where market evaluations are regarded as erroneous (and thus require correction) or where markets do not exist at all and thus imputations of values are required.' Culyer (1976, pp. 66–71) is critical of the 'benefits equals averted costs' approach to benefit evaluation, but this is to some extent misleading because it creates the illusion of a separateness between costs and benefits. What his criticisms are really directed at are those studies that have a very limited notion of what 'averted costs' are, e.g. those studies that, for example, only identify investment-type benefits.
2. Neither of the authors has suffered a broken leg, so C_3 may be wildly displaced.
3. The sum of £3940 was estimated as the economic benefit from preventing the birth of an infant with myelocele (a form of spina bifida). It was estimated that one case (born alive) would be identified in the screened population.
4. Readers unfamiliar with Mr Enoch Powell can substitute the name of their currently most controversial public figure.
5. For purposes of exposition we have presented CBA and CEA as clear-cut alternatives; however, there is a middle position. It is possible to construct hybrid studies with financial outcomes measured as far as possible and other outcomes measured in physical terms and hence placed on the cost–benefit balance, albeit in an awkward manner.

REFERENCES

Bacon, R. and Eltis, W. (1976) *Britain's Economic Problem: Too Few Producers*, Basingstoke and London: Macmillan.

Blaug, M. (1970) *An Introduction to the Economics of Education*. Harmondsworth: Penguin.

COMMITTEE ON CHRONIC KIDNEY DISEASE (1967) *Report*, Washington DC: Bureau of the Budget.

COOPER, M. H. and CULYER, A. J. (ed.) (1973) *Health Economics*. Harmondsworth: Penguin.

CULYER, A. J. (1971) 'The Nature of the Commodity "Health Care" and its Efficient Allocation', *Oxford Economic Papers*, Vol. 23, No. 2 (July), pp. 1891–1211; reprinted as Reading 2 in Cooper and Culyer (1973).

CULYER, A. J. (1976) *Need and the National Health Service*. London: Martin Robertson.

CULYER, A. J., LAVERS, R. J. and WILLIAMS, A. (1971) 'Social Indicators: Health', *Social Trends*, No. 2, pp. 31–42.

CURRIE, J. M., MURPHY, J. A. and SCHMITZ, A. (1971) 'The Concepts of Surplus and its use in Economic Analysis', *Economic Journal*, Vol. 81, No. 324 (December), pp. 741–99.

DASGUPTA, A. K. and PEARCE, D. W. (1972) *Cost – Benefit Analysis: Theory and Practice*. London and Basingstoke: Macmillan.

DOLL, R. (1974) *To Measure N.H.S. Progress* (Somerville Hastings Memorial Lecture, Fabian Occasional Paper 8). London: Fabian Society.

DOWIE, J. A. (1970) 'Valuing the Benefits of Health Improvement', *Australian Economic Papers*, Vol. 9, No. 14 (June), pp. 21–41.

DRAPER, P. and SMART, T. (1974) 'Social Science and Health Policy in the United Kingdom: Some Contributions of the Social Sciences to the Bureaucratization of the National Health Service', *International Journal of Health Services*, Vol. 4, No. 3, (Summer), pp. 453–70.

DROR, Y. (1967) 'Policy Analysts: A New Professional Role in Government Service', *Public Administration Review*, Vol. 27, No. 3 (September), pp. 197–203.

DRUMMOND, M. F. (1977) 'Evaluation and the National Health Service'; paper submitted to the Royal Commission on the National Health Service, January, and published, pp. 67–83, in Culyer, A. J. and Wright, K. G. (eds), *Economic Aspects of Health Services*. London: Martin Robertson.

FANSHEL, S. and BUSH, J. W. (1970) 'A Health Status Index and Its Application to Health Service's Outcomes', *Operations Research*, Vol. 18, No. 6 (November–December), pp. 1021–66.

FORSTER, D. P. (1977) 'A Survey of Obstetric Practice in the Trent Region in Relation to the Prevention of Down's Syndrome', *Public Health*, Vol. 91, pp. 179–82.

GLASS, N. J. (1973) 'Cost – benefit Analysis and Health Services', *Health Trends*, Vol. 5 (August), pp. 51–6.

HAGARD, S. and CARTER, F. A. (1976) 'Preventing the Birth of Infants with Down's Syndrome: A Cost Benefit Analysis', *British Medical Journal*, Vol. 1, No. 6012 (27 March), pp. 753–6.

HOBBS, J. T. (1974) 'Surgery and Sclerotherapy in the Treatment of Varicose Veins', *Archives of Surgery*, Vol. 109 (December), pp. 793–6.

JONES-LEE, M. W., (1976) *The Value of Life: An Economic Analysis*. London: Martin Robertson.

KAMERSCHEN, D. R. and VALENTINE, L. M. (1977), *Intermediate Microeconomic Theory*. Cincinnati, Ohio: South Western Publishing Co.

KLARMAN, H. E. (1965) 'Syphilis Control Programmes' pp. 367–414. In Dorfman, R. (ed.) *Measuring Benefits of Government Investments*. Washington DC: The Brookings Institution.

KLARMAN, H. E. (1974) 'Application of Cost Benefit Analysis to Health Services and the Special Case of Technologic Innovation', *International Journal of Health Services*, Vol. 4, No. 2 (Spring), pp. 325–52.

KLARMAN, H. E., FRANCIS, J. O'S. and ROSENTHAL, G. D. (1968) 'Cost Effectiveness Analysis Applied to the Treatment of Chronic Renal Disease', *Medical Care*, Vol. 6, No. 1 (January/February), pp. 48–54; reprinted as Reading 8 in Cooper and Culyer (1973).

MCKEAN, R. N. (1965) 'The Unseen Hand in Government', *American Economic Review*, Vol. 55, No. 3 (June), pp. 496–506.

MEEK, R. L. (1972) *Figuring out Society*. London: Fontana/Collins.

MISHAN, E. J. (1975) *Cost – Benefit Analysis*, 2nd edn. London: George Allen & Unwin.

MUSGRAVE, R. A. and MUSGRAVE, P. B. (1976) *Public Finance in Theory and Practice*, 2nd edn. New York: McGraw-Hill.

PEACOCK, A. T. and WISEMAN, J. (1966) Economic Growth and the Principles of Educational Finance in Developed Countries, pp. 89–99 in *Financing of Education for Economic Growth*. Paris: O.E.C.D.

PIACHAUD, D. and WEDDELL, J. M. (1972) 'The Economics of Treating Varicose Veins', *International Journal of Epidemiology*, Vol. 1, No. 3, pp. 287–94.

POLE, D. (1971) 'Mass Radiography: A Cost Benefit Approach', pp. 45–56 in McLachlan, G. (ed.) *Problems and Progress in Medical Care* (5th Series). London: Oxford University Press for the Nuffield Provincial Hospitals Trust.

ROBERTS, J. A. (1974) 'Economic Evaluation of Health Care', *British Journal of Preventive and Social Medicine*, Vol. 28, No. 3 (August), pp. 210–16.

ROBINSON, D. (1971) Cost and Effectiveness of a Program to Prevent Rheumatic Fever', *Health Services and Mental Health Administration*, Health Reports, Vol. 18, No. 3 (April), pp. 385–9.

ROSSER, R. M. and WATTS, V. C. (1972) 'The Measurement of Hospital Output', *International Journal of Epidemiology*, Vol. 1, No. 4, pp. 361–7.

SELF, P. (1970) 'Nonsense on Stilts: The Futility of Roskill', *Political Quarterly*, Vol. 41, No. 3 (July), pp. 249–60: reprinted in *New Society*, Vol. 16, No. 405 (2 July 1970), pp. 8–11.

STEINER, P. O. (1974) 'Public Expenditure Budgeting', pp. 241–357 in Blinder, A. S. *et al.*, *The Economics of Public Finance*. Washington, DC: Brookings Institution.

WAGER, R. (1972) *Care of the Elderly*. London: Institute of Municipal Treasurers and Accountants.

WARD, R. A. (1975) *The Economics of Health Resources*. Reading, Massachusetts: Addison-Wesley.

WEISBROD, B. A. (1968) 'Income Redistribution Effects and Benefit Cost Analysis', pp. 177–209 in Chase, S. B. Jr (ed.) *Problems in Public Expenditure Analysis*. Washington DC: Brookings Institution.

WILLIAMS, A. (1972) 'Cost – Benefit Analysis: Bastard Science? and/or Insidious Poison in the Body Politik?' *Journal of Public Economics*, Vol. 1, No. 2 (August), pp. 199–225.

WILLIAMS, A. (1974) 'The Cost Benefit Approach', *British Medical Bulletin*, Vol. 30, No. 3 (September), pp. 252–6.

WILLIAMS, A. (1978) 'Income Distribution and Public Expenditure Decisions', Chapter 5, pp. 65–80 in Posner, M. V. (ed.), *Public Expenditure*. Cambridge: University Press.

WILLIAMS, A. and ANDERSON, R. (1975) *Efficiency in the Social Services*. Oxford: Basil Blackwell; London: Martin Robertson.

WRIGHT, K. G. (1974) 'Alternative Measures of the Output of Social Programmes: The Elderly', pp. 239–72 in Culyer, A. J. (ed.) (1974) *Economic Policies and Social Goals: Aspects of Public Choice*. London: Martin Robertson.

9 Valuing Human Life

> Death is an awesome and indivisible event that goes but once to a customer in a single large size.
>
> *T. C. Schelling* (1968, p. 158)

9.1 Introduction

One of the benefits associated with many health and indeed other projects is the saving of human life. If cost–benefit analysis is to be a useful guide to resource allocation decisions, a satisfactory method of placing a value on this benefit must be found. Luckily for the policy analyst, this is one area of health economics that has attracted the attention of many economists, through both theoretical and empirical work. In the discussion below an attempt is made to group the various contributions around particular approaches to this emotive issue. In the final section a brief answer to the question, 'which method is right?' is suggested. The approaches analysed are placed under heads suggested by Acton (1973, p. 62):

(a) livelihood or human capital-based measures;
(b) valuations implicit in past decisions;
(c) valuations that are derived from individualistic behaviour in the market or more directly elicited measures of willingness to pay (WTP).

Acton also introduced a fourth category, 'explicit statements of politically designated persons'. He dismissed this approach largely because 'it is hard to find politically designated persons who will state the buying price of reduced mortality' (Acton, 1973, p. 62). It is however worth noting, as it follows on Williams's (1974) notion that a given stated value could be given to a health 'point' and then its value become part of the political and government process rising (presumably) over time at a rate depending on the extent of its popularity with the voters. A similar process could in principle be followed with human life valuation. The government could choose a starting value, say the lowest life value currently implicit in government decisions, and then let the value be a political issue, to be put to the voters in election manifestos.

In the discussion that follows two interrelated issues need to be borne in mind. First, what is the purpose for which the value of a life is required? One method of valuing life may make more sense in one context than in another. Second, are the people whose lives are to be valued currently alive? If they are not, then we are in an *ex post* situation valuing the lost life of, inevitably, a *known* individual. If the situation is the *ex ante* one, then it is generally assumed that we do not know the identity of the individual whose life is at stake and to be valued. This latter distinction between *ex ante* and *ex post* calculations has featured prominantly in the literature on human life valuation although its relevance has very recently been challenged. However, before evaluating life-valuing techniques, the techniques themselves must be outlined.

9.2 Livelihood or human capital-based measures

The earliest attempts at valuing a human life concerned themselves with the capital value of a man. Apart from the slave traders, the first person to calculate the average value of a human being was Sir William Petty in the late eighteenth century. It is worth noting the purpose of his calculations, since it is argued here that the appropriate method of valuing life depends on what it is hoped will be achieved. Kiker (1966) has argued that Petty used the notion to:

(a) demonstrate the power of England;
(b) indicate the economic effects of migration;
(c) establish the money value of human life destroyed by war;
(d) establish the monetary loss to a nation resulting from deaths.

The way in which Petty estimated the value of the stock of human capital was to capitalise the wage bill to perpetuity using the market rate of interest. The wage bill was derived by subtracting profits and rents from national income. Dublin and Lotka (1930) summarise Petty's approach in the formula:

$$L = Y_l/i$$

where L is the value of human capital, Y_l is the annual income of labour and i is the discount rate (5 per cent).

Kiker (1966) indicated that Petty was not alone in treating human beings and their skills as capital. Two basic methods were used: the capitalised earnings approach outlined above, and the cost of production approach. The latter consisted in trying to estimate the real costs (usually net of maintenance) in 'producing' a human being. In general, the purpose of such calculations was broadened beyond those listed above to include calculations to determine the economic effects of education and health investment, to propose equitable tax schemes, to emphasise the economic value of life and hence health conservation, and finally to aid courts in cases involving compensation for personal injury or death. Our concern here, however, is to consider a selection of more recent contributions to what is clearly not a novel question in economics.

A convenient example of the methodology of the value of livelihood is provided by Rice and Cooper: 'The value of human life *expressed in terms of life time earnings* is a basic tool of the economist, programme planner, government administrator and others who are interested in measuring the social benefits associated with investments in particular programs'[1] (Rice and Cooper, 1967, p. 1954; emphasis ours). Consequently their aim 'is to provide improved, refined, comprehensive and up-to-date estimates of the present value of lifetime earnings in considerable detail according to age, sex, colour and educational level' (Rice and Cooper, 1967, p. 1954). A health care project that reduces mortality in a specific age and colour group can be estimated by use of the lifetime earnings data for that group as a measure of their productive contribution.

Rice and Cooper based their estimates on the following seven assumptions.

Life expectancy. The lifetime earnings data were developed on the assumption that each cohort will follow his or her pattern of life expectancy as for 1964 at successive ages.

Labour force participation. The assumption made here is that an individual will be in the labour force and productive during his expected lifetime in accordance with the current (1965) pattern of labour force participation for his sex, colour and educational level.

Earnings. Estimated mean earnings data adjusted upwards for employer expenditures on workers (e.g. social insurance contributions) were used as the measure of an individual's output.

Housewives' services. These were estimated at the average earnings rate of a domestic worker (1964).

Discounting. The assumed discount rate was 4 per cent (though the sensitivity of the results to other discount rates was also examined).

Productivity increases. To adjust for the gain in productivity (and hence higher earnings) that takes place over time, a nominal discount rate of approximately 7 per cent was then reduced to allow for productivity rises of 3 per cent per annum yielding a net discount rate of approximately 4 per cent (1.07/1.03 = 1.039) – the one used in the study.

Allowance for consumption. Since the individual personally consumes part of his contributions to output, the output gain to the rest of society owing to his presence in the work force is less than his total output. Clearly, if we are considering whether to introduce a health programme that saves life, the consumption of the individual is *ex ante* no different from the consumption by others of his surplus output. Yet if he dies, society (i.e. those who remain alive) has lost only his output net of consumption. Rice and Cooper took the view that they were measuring the economic value of a man and not his value only to others, e.g. his family.

Dawson (1967) extended the methodology while using earnings net of consumption as the base for his calculations. His extensions were designed to take some account of the result that those who are not in the work force have no value attached to their lives by the calculation process (e.g. old-age pensioners.). These include pain and suffering and similar non-production aspects. However, in the absence of accurate measures of these losses, the author used the following values of the subjective cost of casualties:

fatality[2]	£5000
serious casualty	£ 200
slight casualty	£ 0

For a death, e.g. in a road accident, it is the value of the net output plus £5000 that is the appropriate valuation from this methodology.

Mishan (1971) has been particularly critical of the *gross* output approach because it assumes that maximising gross national product is society's objective and that economic changes should be valued by reference to it. The net output approach has been criticised on the grounds that it uses an *ex post* view of society when an *ex ante* view is required. Although these are damaging criticisms, recent contributions to the *Economic Journal* have discussed the British legal system's use of the *ex post* net output criteria. Dawson argued that his approach to fatalities was the one in use in British courts, and it is this process that has been subject of debate. Kidner and Richards (1974) were concerned with the adequacy of compensation in the form of damages for those killed in circumstances that come under the Fatal Accidents Acts 1846–1959. The basic principle in the legislation is one of full compensation, i.e. the total amount the widow would have received from the deceased (paid as a capital sum). The calculation involves three steps: (a) calculation of the period of time the family would have been dependent upon the deceased (normally this would be the latter's expected working life); (b) calculation of the amount of the dependency, i.e. the amount contributed by the husband to the maintenance of the family, that is earnings net of tax and *own consumption*; (c) calculation of the necessary multiplier to capitalise the sum over the period of the dependency. The latter process may be very casual, the judge applying a multiplier to a person of a certain age group based on the experience of previous cases. The idea is that dependants are awarded a capital sum by the judge such that if they spent a sum equal in size to the dependency each year, and if a certain rate of interest (expected by the judge) was earned on the remaining capital each year, the capital sum would just last the estimated period of the dependency. Kidner and Richards criticised the method on several grounds, e.g. the fact that it takes no account of inflation or the increasing real income the deceased would have expected to enjoy. They advocated a 'no fault' system, as in New Zealand, where the dependant normally receives annually 40 per cent of the deceased's pretax earnings plus 13.3 per cent of the earnings for each child up to a total limit of

80 per cent of the earnings. The widow and children in addition receive a capital sum of $1000 and $500 respectively.

The article generated several comments and replies (see Phillips, Hawkins and Flemming, 1975a; Richards and Kidner, 1975; Phillips, Hawkins and Flemming, 1975b; Doherty, Lees and Bates, 1976; and Kidner and Richards, 1976) which cast further doubts on the existing process of calculating appropriate compensatory sums in Britain. Unfortunately, little or no attention was directed to the question of what ought to be the basis of compensation. However, there was general agreement that an 'open and systematic approach' was desirable.

In sharp contrast to the British experience, courts in the United States have awarded dependents sums greatly in excess of expected earnings. However, the desire to punish the negligent party (and claim back any profits made from the negligence) may be as strong a motive as the compensation of the family for pain and grief over and above loss of income.

9.3 Valuation implicit in past decisions

Before surveying life valuation attempts under this heading it is useful to distinguish two types of implicit values:

(a) implicit values that derive from political, administrative or other processes that do not reflect in any real way the views or decisions of the individual whose life is being valued;

(b) implicit values that derive from individual decisions about compensation for risk of death, e.g. pay premiums in hazardous jobs. These valuations have a lot in common with the WTP approach but are found lacking as acceptable WTP measures when analysed in detail. For this reason they have been included under this heading rather than the one below.

9.3.1 Implicit values from the decisions of others

Looking at valuations that are implicit in decisions made not by individuals but by persons of authority on their behalf has been popular with some analysts. If, for example, an air force pilot is lost at sea and the plane is known to be a 'write-off' with no scrap value, and the air force authorities devote four days of eight pilots' time and the navy devotes three ship-days to finding the pilot before calling off the search, the real resource value of the men and machines used in the search could be interpreted as the minimum value put on saving a life. Sinclair (1969) provides a more concrete example of this approach in discussing the introduction of British legislation to make cabs on farm tractors compulsory. He argued that the home market in Britain for tractors was 100,000 per annum. With an average five-year life per tractor, all British farm tractors would have cabs within a five-year period, saving about forty lives per annum over the period. The cost of the cabs was £200 million (£40 per cab), and with 200 lives saved over the five years the implicit value of a tractor driver's life is £100,000. (We are grateful to Mooney, 1977, for drawing our attention to this example.)

The fundamental problem with this approach is that the economist is using the air force/naval authorities and the legislator to do his job for him. In general, although this type of approach has a superficial plausibility and is often ingenious, it is not consistent with the economist's approach. However, this implicit valuation approach is not without policy relevance. Where implicit valuations of life vary widely over different public sector activities and where concern is with the saving of life *per se*, resources should be allocated in a cost-effective way. If for example it turns out that the value of a life in the construction industry is £10,000 in the sense that the expenditure of £10,000 on improved safety saves one life, whereas it costs £2000 worth of resources to save a life by providing safer playgrounds for children, it is rational to devote any life-saving budget to the latter until the marginal cost of saving an additional life is equalised in all activities. (For some actual valuations of life implicit in policy, see Mooney, 1977, Appendix C.)

9.3.2 Implicit values from individual decisions

Individuals often trade off increased risk of death against increased personal compensation, e.g. steeplejacks and oil rig fire-fighters. Fromm (1965) argued that, by dividing the measure of increased compensation by the change in the probability of death, the value of life can be established. That is, if a steeplejack is paid (and accepts) an additional £2000 per year for the hazardous rating of his job and faces a differential probability of death at work of 0.01, then he implicitly values his life at £2000/0.01 = £200,000. Reversing one of Fromm's examples will serve to re-emphasise this approach. In 1962, among 54.9 million passengers carried over 34,710 passenger-miles on American domestic routes, there were 158 deaths in 5 accidents. Excluding 37 deaths due to dynamite sabotage, there were 0.34 deaths per million passenger-miles; and, with an assumed median trip length of 500 miles, the probability of dying per trip was approximately 0.00017 per cent. If individuals were prepared to pay 68 cents per trip to reduce that probability to zero, then the implied values of their lives would be $0.68/0.0000017 or $400,000. The approach has also been used recently by Melinek (1974) to produce a series of calculations using data from the use of pedestrian subways, smoking and hazardous job pay differentials. These approaches have been criticised (Mishan, 1971) however because of the implied linearity assumption of the relationship between the probability of death and the WTP to reduce that probability. Does it make sense to suppose that, because an individual will accept £200 to compensate him for an increased risk of death from 0.001 to 0.002, he would accept £200,000 for the probability to move from zero to one? A further criticism is that frequently individuals may be totally unaware of the small probability differences involved. Are workers aware of the risks of different types of occupation and the pay differentials associated with them? A drawback to using insurance data is that life insurance is purchased to compensate one's family in the event of death, not oneself. For further reservations to this type of approach see Rhoads (1978).

9.4 Valuations derived from individuals' preferences (WTP)

Mishan (1971), drawing on the work of Schelling (1968), has made a valuable contribution to the debate over human life valuation by pointing out that economists already had a mechanism for evaluating changes in economic welfare, namely the compensating variation discussed in Chapter 8, and asking why this approach should not be applied to loss of life or limb. At first sight the approach may seem inappropriate. If someone loses his life as the result of the introduction of a particular project, then the compensating variation (CV) measures the minimum sum he would be prepared to accept in order to put up with the project[3] that results in his death! Well, not quite. Mishan's second insight was to emphasise that the appropriate CVs should be evaluated *ex ante* rather than *ex post*. The importance of the distinction is that *ex ante* all that is known is that an additional person in the relevant population is to die, but not which person. Therefore the CVs would measure the minimum sum that the individuals would accept to put up with an increased *probability* of their death that results from the introduction of the project.

An example makes the approach clear. Suppose 1000 local people are affected by the building of a new isolation hospital for contagious diseases in a remote village, and the expectation is that as a consequence of some accident at the hospital there will be one death in the coming period. The villagers are affected to the extent that there is an increased expectation of death for each one of them of 1 in 1000, or 0.001. When carrying out the CBA of the isolation hospital there will be included on the negative side the CVs corresponding to this decrease in welfare. By summing the CVs associated with this probability of one additional death, a value of life has been generated. But it must be remembered that it is not derived as the value put on the certain death of a given individual but reflects the compensation required by the villagers in return for bearing the increased *risk* of death.

A further refinement in the treatment of risk is required, however, because not all risks are of the same kind. Mishan has proposed a classification of risk according to two characteristics. *Direct* risks are risks of one's own death, whereas *indirect* risks are those risks that arise from one's concern (financial or psychic) with the risks to the rest of society. *Voluntary* risks are accepted by individuals, *involuntary* risks are forced upon them. Table 9.1 outlines the possibilities discussed by Mishan. Risk R^1 is the direct voluntary risk. Here the concern is with the acquisition of a product or service that directly affects the probability of death, for example a car. Because people know that car-driving increases the risk of their death, such risks are evaluated by the jth consumer at an amount r^1_{jj} at the time of the decision, e.g. buying a new car, and are subtracted from the riskless consumer surplus, C_j, expected from driving a new car. If the individual is observed to go ahead and purchase the car then $C_j - r^1_{jj} > 0$.

Table 9.1 Mishan's Risk Classification

Risk type	For individual j Risk from own-risk exposure	Risk from others' actions or risk exposure	For society $j = 1 \ldots n$
Voluntary direct R^1	r^1_{jj}	$\sum_{i=1}^{n} r^1_{ij} \quad (i \neq j)$	including j in i and subtracting from the consumer surplus of driving (C_j) $\sum_{j=1}^{n}\left(C_j - \sum_{i=1}^{n} r^1_{ij}\right)$ gives consumer surplus from driving net of risk
Involuntary direct R^2	r^2_{jj}	$\sum_{i=1}^{n} r^2_{ij} \quad (i \neq j)$	including j in i and summing to give the community CVs $\sum_{j=1}^{n}\sum_{i=1}^{n} r^2_{ij}$
Financial involuntary direct R^3	—	$\sum_{i=1}^{n} r^3_{ij} \quad (i \neq j)$	excluding j from i and summing to give the community CVs $\sum_{j=1}^{n}\sum_{i=1}^{n} r^3_{ij} \quad (i \neq j)$
Psychic involuntary indirect R^4	—	$\sum_{i=1}^{n} r^4_{ij} \quad (i \neq j)$	excluding j from i and summing to give the community CVs $\sum_{j=1}^{n}\sum_{i=1}^{n} r^4_{ij} \quad (i \neq j)$

It must be remembered that the risk the car-driver faces varies directly with the number of other car-drivers on the road. Therefore there is a second risk compensation sum that j must net out, r^1_{ij}, the sum required to compensate him for the risk he is put to by other drivers. Individuals can avoid both risks by not driving. Therefore if they drive it can only be concluded that the consumer surplus, net of risk compensations of both types, remains positive; i.e.,

$$\left(C_j - \sum_{i=1}^{n} r^1_{ij}\right) > 0$$

(when $i = j$, the self-imposed risk, is included.). Aggregating over the n-person community gives

$$\sum_{j=1}^{n} \left(C_j - \sum_{i=1}^{n} r_{ij}^1 \right)$$

as the consumer surplus benefit net of the voluntary direct risks of driving for car-drivers. Evaluation of a new car plant therefore can safely ignore such risks. They have, in effect, been 'capitalised' by the market.

All remaining types of risk are assumed involuntarily and as a consequence need to be taken account of in CBA. Involuntary direct risks (R^2) are risks to the individual that come from, e.g., the reprocessing of UK and foreign nuclear waste at Windscale. This is a primary risk and can in principle be compensated by the sum $r_{jj}{}^2$. There is also the secondary risk that some affected individual will pass the contamination on to you. The compensation sum appropriate to this secondary direct involuntary risk is termed $r_{ij}{}^2$ ($i \neq j$). Summing the risks for the whole community and including j within i (he runs some risk if he is the sole inhabitant) yields

$$\sum_{j=1}^{n} \sum_{i=1}^{n} r_{ij}^2 .$$

Indirect risks flow from concern with others. The financial aspect (R^3) arises because on balance the death of an individual, i, will improve or hurt j's financial position. Hence if an additional chance of i's death involves the possibility of financial improvement for j, the CV associated with this risk, r^3ij, will be positive. Conversely, if i's death would reduce j's income, r^3ij would be negative. For individual j's financial connections with the rest of society the sum of the relevant CVs is

$$\sum_{i=1}^{n} r_{ij}^3 \qquad i \neq j.$$

For the whole community the sum becomes

$$\sum_{j=1}^{n} \sum_{i=1}^{n} r_{ij}^3 \qquad i \neq j.$$

(As with R^4 below j is excluded from i by definition.) The final category of risk (R^4) is also involuntary and indirect as is R^3, but is concerned with possible psychic costs and benefits derived from the death of others. For most individuals it seems safe to assume that, the greater the risks others are exposed to, the more their own welfare is reduced, so that the CV needed to compensate for increased risks of death of others, especially friends and relatives, is positive; i.e.,

$$\sum_{i=1}^{n} r_{ij}^{4} > 0 \qquad i \neq j.$$

For the community as a whole the sum of CVs generated because of the psychic motive are given by:

$$\sum_{j=1}^{n} \sum_{i=1}^{n} r_{ij}^{4} \qquad i \neq j.$$

R^2, R^3 and R^4 are the relevant CVs to be used in cost–benefit analysis to evaluate any expected saving or loss of life. R^1 is ignored because it is accepted voluntarily and thus must have been included in individuals' calculations at some point.

Mishan anticipated complications in operationalising his approach and envisaged the use of 'data yielded by surveys based on the questionnaire method' (Mishan, 1971, p. 705), and justified his overall approach with the oft-quoted words 'that there is more to be said for rough estimates of the precise concept than precise estimates of economically irrelevant concepts' (Mishan, 1971, p. 705). Economically irrelevant concepts would include all those discussed earlier in this chapter.

The probability basis for valuing life via the amount individuals would pay to enjoy a reduction in their probability of death is currently widely accepted as the correct theoretical method. Jones-Lee (1969), (also see Jones-Lee, 1974, 1976) has used it to identify the amount an individual would pay to avoid certain death by road accident as a special case where the probability of death changes from 0 to 1. With the aid of a Von Neumann–Morgenstern utility experiment, he estimated how much an individual would pay to secure a reduction in the probability of his own death, by confronting the test person with a series of hypothetical choices between different 'states of the world' involving various probabilities of his own death (by road accident) and the enjoyment of an income of £10,000 per annum and no work. Acton (1973) has conveniently reduced such WTP approaches

Lottery A		*Lottery B*
Comprises a p chance of $U(D, W)$ and $(1-p)$ chance of $U(L, W)$	$\sim$	Comprises a $p\text{-}\Delta p$ chance of $U(D, W\text{-}V)$ and $(1-p+\Delta p)$ chance of $U(L, W\text{-}V)$

Figure 9.1 *Willingness to pay for a reduction in the probability of death per time period*

to their essence. The test individual can be confronted with choices between the health status being alive (L for living) and dead (D) and wealth level (W). In any given time period he faces a probability of dying, p, but is assumed able to purchase a reduction in that probability, Δp. The question is, what is the maximum purchase price (V) he will pay in order to secure the decrease in the probability of his death? The possibilities are summarised in Figure 9.1. The sum V is an amount such that he will be indifferent between two lotteries giving expected utility $E(U_A)$ and $E(U_B)$ such that

$$E(U_A) = p \cdot U(D, W) + (1-p)U(L, W) \tag{9.1}$$

$$E(U_B) = (p-\Delta p)U(D, W-V) + (1-p+\Delta p)U(L, W-V) \tag{9.2}$$

and

$$E(U_A) = E(U_B). \tag{9.3}$$

That is, the expected utility from facing probability (p) of death and $(1-p)$ of life with wealth (W) must equal that from facing the reduced probability of death with lower wealth. (N.B. Wealth left to descendants does not necessarily carry zero utility *ex ante*.)

9.5 Some uses and reservations

Criticisms of the livelihood and implicit value approaches were introduced in the discussions above, but this is not to imply the approaches are useless. There is some role for both of them. If one is seeking to calculate the rate of return in the sense of the contribution to economic growth of resources devoted to health care (see Section 2.2.2) or to compensate the next of kin for the loss of the 'breadwinner' aspect of the spouse, then the discounted value of future earnings seems a relevant magnitude to begin with at least. The first type of implicit value approach, as indicated, makes it clear how life-saving resources can be employed in a cost-effective way, which is clearly valuable information.

As regards the WTP approach, this has widespread support as *the* way to value human life in public policy appraisal. But criticisms of it have been voiced by some who feel it is not as sound a method of human life evaluation as supposed. One reservation concerning the approach based on WTP for small changes in probability of death remains unresolved. This is that consumers typically do not make their choices in terms of probabilities but in terms of certainties. This may be particularly important where life and death are concerned. A probability of winning a lottery conveys some impression of the expected financial outcome if the lottery is played repeatedly. But the expected outcome of life or death is intangible. In the long run you cannot be 20 per cent dead and in the short run you are either alive or dead. Not only are individuals unaccustomed to making such decisions, but also they are likely to behave based on their subjective evaluation of the outcome.[4] Individuals can, and frequently do, convince themselves that average probabilities of death do not apply to them in order to rationalise their actions (e.g. 'I never wear a seat belt because I am a safe driver'). Alternatively, they may take a fatalist view: death results from a series of interacting factors and will happen regardless of any minor adjustments in behaviour (e.g. 'if I'm going to have a serious accident anyway, a seat belt won't make much difference'). Finally, consumers are used to buying an increased range of products that have guarantees attached. No such guaranteed outcome is offered when paying for a small reduction in the probability of death, and so consumers may be reluctant to offer more than a trivial sum. Thus, a dying individual may be prepared to pay for an operation that might save his life but we would argue that this amount would be unlikely to vary with small changes in the probability of success. Either the individual expects (or, more accurately, hopes) that it will save his life or he thinks it hopeless. It may be argued that consumers make sensible choices only after learning from experience; e.g., note the disappointment of children when a toy or meal *they* have chosen fails to provide the anticipated pleasure. They have to learn. But there is no scope for learning when buying reductions in the probability of death. If in doubt, try deciding for yourself the value of the safety belt fitted to your car. Then look up the accident figures and see what effect the belt has on the probability of your staying alive. Did you value it too high or too low?

In part these are the concerns raised by Fromm (1977). Fromm argues the WTP approaches[5] to the valuation of injury and mortality reduction when summed only serve to establish a floor and not a ceiling for values that could be deemed to arise from social preferences, for several reasons.

(a) The expected value of a given life-saving programme to an individual could proportionately be far less than for the population as a whole. Using Fromm's example, if the death rate of the U.S. male population is 1 per cent and from major cardiovascular disease is approximately 0.5 per cent, and the latter could be reduced by 20 per cent by a new procedure, then the expected pay-off to the individual is $(0.005)(0.20)U(V)$ where $U(V)$ is the utility of life. Since without the procedure the individual has a 99 per cent chance of living and with it 99.1 per cent, an improvement of 0.1 per cent, he might well conclude it is not worth the certain loss of paying for the procedure for the possibility that the procedure would be useful to him. After all, he may well feel he stood a far greater chance of death from other causes before heart disease might affect him. However, can the government also treat these potential life saving gains as being valueless?

(b) There may be very little variance in the population probability of death but substantial variance for individual probabilities; i.e., no assurance can be given to any individual that he will benefit from a particular life-saving programme, and hence willingness to pay might be very low. For the whole population however the number and average characteristics of individuals who would benefit can be predicted with near certainty, and again government policy makers should weigh this information in their calculations irrespective of any willingness to pay.

(c) A point that could have equally well been made in Chapter 8 relates to the role of income distribution in the CBA/WTP approach. A moment's reflection makes it clear that individual compensating variations for changes in the probability of death or any other change will by and large vary directly with individual *ability* to pay; i.e., CBA, in the simple form outlined in Chapter 8, takes the distribution of income as a given, and hence (as always!) the rich are in a more favoured position. In the value of life debate this point is more readily appreciated, as many believe that, in something so basic as life/death-affecting decisions, the rich and the poor should be afforded the means of an 'equal say'.

The most savage attack on the WTP approach has come from Broome (1978), who has argued that the whole approach is bogus in that it relies on ignorance to make it work. It is agreed by all commentators that an individual would not accept any finite sum for the certain loss of his life, and hence in Broome's view CBA is not operational on a project that involves a death. Broome is well aware that ignorance of who is going to die can transform the calculation and make an *ex ante* valuation of a lost life possible, as discussed in Section 9.4. However, is this acceptable? Broome's answer is 'no', his reasoning being that CBA and the *ex ante* evaluation of investment projects is a relevant technique only if it is an accurate reflection of the *ex post* realised situation. With a lost human life in the *ex post* situation this is clearly not the case, as the *ex ante* calculation would have to incorporate a negative infinitely large sum and the NPV of the project could never be positive. This is not to imply that all projects involving a death cannot represent an improvement in welfare, but rather that CBA cannot evaluate them as such.

It is clear that WTP approaches to human life valuation are not without difficulties. More generally, Fromm concludes that

> All methods of specifying or estimating life and injury values to be used in benefit–cost studies of changes in safety regulations and other life-prolonging programmes have serious imperfections, and far more research in this area is needed. [Fromm, 1977, pp. 18–19]

9.6 Summary

This chapter has surveyed attempts to put a value on human life. The various contributions have been collected under three headings – the livelihood approach, the implicit value approach and the WTP approach. Of these it is generally claimed that the third is superior from the economist's (CBA) viewpoint, as it puts the loss or saving of life on the same footing as all other costs and benefits, all being measured by reference to individual compensating variations. However, this is not universally accepted, as indicated in the last section. It was also argued that the value of life will vary to some extent with the decision-making context and the purpose for which a value of life is required.

Given the difficulties surrounding the probability method and the need for further research, we would argue that in the meantime consistency, as opposed to hysterical reaction, is required for public policy towards life-saving investment, and that such values as exist implicitly should be brought out for explicit discussion. Then, at very least, it will be possible to ensure that similar values of life are being used to evaluate public projects without systematic biases in particular safety areas such as road safety or health.

NOTES

1. This approach is sexist to the extent that in general males have higher lifetime earnings than females and are hence of greater value.
2. The figure for the fatality is derived from the minimum value implied by the fact that society is prepared to support old-age pensioners who have a negative net output. Since society is prepared to support an old-age pensioner whose estimated net output has a discounted present value of £5000, the value of the subjective cost of his death must be at least £5000.
3. It is possible for even this approach to yield a sensible *minimum* valuation. See Akehurst and Culyer (1974).
4. For a very amusing discussion that relates to death and people's perceptions of probabilities see Lisa Alther's best-seller *Kinflicks*. In the early pages the author writes about Ginny's (the heroine's) fear of dying while flying and continues: 'Ginny had often thought that she should carry . . . a bomb aboard her plane flights herself, because the likelihood of there being *two* bomb-toting psychopaths on the same flight was so infinitesimal as to be an impossibility' (Alther, 1977, p. 14).
5. Defined as the monetary equivalent of explicit, implicit or imputed individual preferences for injury or mortality reduction.

REFERENCES

ACTON, J. P. (1973) *Evaluating Public Programmes to Save Lives: The Case of Heart Attacks*. Santa Monica, California: Rand Corporation.

AKEHURST, R. L. and CULYER, A. J. (1974) 'On the Economic Surplus and the Value of Life', *Bulletin of Economic Research*, Vol. 26, No. 2 (November), pp. 63–78.

ALTHER, L. (1977) *Kinflicks*, Harmondsworth: Penguin.

BROOME, J. (1978) 'Trying to Value a Life', *Journal of Public Economics*, Vol. 9, No. 1 (February), pp. 91–100.

COOPER, M. H. and CULYER, A. J. (eds) (1973) *Health Economics*. Harmondsworth: Penguin.

DAWSON, R. F. F. (1967) *Cost of Road Accidents in Great Britain*, Road Research Laboratory, Ministry of Transport, an excerpt from which comprises Reading 14 in Cooper and Culyer (1973).

DAWSON, R. F. F. (1971) *Current Cost of Road Accidents in Great Britain*. Road Research Laboratory, Department of the Environment.

DOHERTY, N., LEES, D., and BATES, J. (1976) 'Compensation to the Dependents of Accident Victims – A Comment', *Economic Journal*, Vol. 86, No. 341 (March), pp. 98–103.

DOWIE, J. A. (1970) 'Valuing the Benefits of Health Improvement', *Australian Economic Papers*, Vol. 9, No. 14 (June), pp. 12–41.

DUBLIN, L. I. and LOTKA, A. J. (1930) *The Money Value of a Man*. New York: Ronald Press; revised edition 1946.

FROMM, G. (1965) 'Civil Aviation Expenditures', pp. 172–230 in Dorfman, R. (ed.), *Measuring Benefits of Government Investments*. Washington DC: Brookings Institution.

FROMM, G. (1977) 'Individual and Social Preferences, Safety Regulations and Life and Injury Valuation', *Rivista Internazionale di Economic adi Transport*, Vol. 4, No. 1, pp. 3–20.

JONES-LEE, M. W. (1969) 'Valuation of Reduction in Probability of Death by Road Accident', *Journal of Transport Economics and Policy*, Vol. 3, No. 1 (January), pp. 37–47; reprinted as Reading 13 in Cooper and Culyer (1973).

JONES-LEE, M. W. (1974) 'The Value of Changes in the Probability of Death or Injury', *Journal of Political Economy*, Vol. 82, No. 4 (July/August), pp. 835–49.

JONES-LEE, M. W. (1976) *The Value of Life: An Economic Analysis*. London: Martin Robertson.

KIDNER, R. and RICHARDS, K. (1974) 'Compensation to Dependants of Accident Victims', *Economic Journal*, Vol. 84, No. 333 (March), pp. 130–42.

KIDNER, R. and RICHARDS, K. (1976) 'Compensation to Dependants of Accident Victims – A Reply', *Economic Journal*, Vol. 86, No. 341 (March), pp. 104–06.

KIKER, B. F. (1966) 'The Historical Roots of the Concept of Human Capital', *Journal of Political Economy*, Vol. 74, No. 5 (October), pp. 481–99; reprinted as reading 1 in Wystra, R. A. (ed.) (1971) *Human Capital Formation and Manpower Development*. New York: Free Press.

LAYARD, R. (ed.) (1972) *Cost Benefit Analysis*. Harmondsworth: Penguin.

MELINEK, S. J. (1974) 'A Method of Evaluating Human Life for Economic Purposes', *Accident Analysis and Prevention*, Vol. 6, No. 3 (October), pp. 103–14.

MISHAN, E. (1971) 'Evaluation of Life and Limb, A Theoretical Approach', *Journal of Political Economy*, Vol. 79, No. 4 (July/August), pp. 687–705; also reprinted as Reading 8 in Layard (1972).

MOONEY, G. H. (1977) *The Valuation of Human Life*. London and Basingstoke: Macmillan.

PHILLIPS, J., HAWKINS, K. and FLEMMING, J. (1975a) 'Compensation for Personal Injuries', *Economic Journal*, Vol. 85, No. 337 (March), pp. 129–34.

PHILLIPS, J., HAWKINS, K. and FLEMMING, J. (1975b) 'Compensation for Personal Injuries – A Reply', *Economic Journal*, Vol. 85, No. 338 (June), pp. 392–4.

RHOADS, S. (1978) 'How Much Should We Spend to Save a Life?' *The Public Interest*, No. 51 (Spring), pp. 74–92.

RICE, D. P. and COOPER, B. S. (1967) 'The Economic Value of Human Life', *American Journal of Public Health*, Vol. 57, No. 11 (November), pp. 1954–6.

RICHARDS, K. and KIDNER, R. (1975) 'Compensation for Personal Injuries – A Comment', *Economic Journal*, Vol. 85, No. 338 (June), pp. 389–92.

SCHELLING, T. C. (1968) 'The Life You Save May Be Your Own', pp. 127–62 in Chase, S. B. Jr (ed.) *Problems in Public Expenditure Analysis*. Washington DC: Brookings Institution, an excerpt from which comprises Reading 12 in Cooper and Culyer (1973).

SINCLAIR, C. (1969) 'Costing the Hazards of Technology', *New Scientist*, Vol. 44, No. 671 (16 October), pp. 120–2.

WILLIAMS, A. (1974) 'Measuring the Effectiveness of Health Care Systems', *British Journal of Preventive and Social Medicine*, Vol. 28, No. 3 (August), pp. 196–202 and pp. 361–76 in Perlman, M. (ed.) (1974) *The Economics of Health and Medical Care*. London and Basingstoke: Macmillan Press for International Economic Association.

PART V
Health Care Policy Problems

10 Economic Aspects of a Public Health Care System: the UK

> In the investigations I had to make for this report, everytime I had scratched through the mud and moss of the overt and vocal signs of unrest, I came down on a solid bedrock of support at all levels for what Aneurin Bevan had introduced in 1946 – the British National Health Service. It is that, more than anything else, that makes me think the NHS – however serious its present problems – will survive not only its 30th birthday, but well into the next century.
>
> *D. Nowlan* (1977, p. 1178)

10.1 Introduction

In this chapter and the two that follow we examine some of the economic problems generated by particular systems of provision of health care. Of necessity we limit discussion to a small set of specific problems thrown up by public, private and developing health care systems. But our choice of issues is not arbitrary. The policy problems of each system are not only of current interest but are to a substantial degree specific to their particular context. Thus, in a system such as the UK's where the greater part of health care is provided free of charge it is not the inflation of costs but the rationing and queueing problems of non-price allocation and the persistence of inequality in a system set up to eradicate it that are seen as major difficulties. Conversely, in the United States, where a substantial proportion of health care services are sold to the consumer, albeit with the frequent intrusion of third party payment from insurance, and where equality has not been an overt goal, price inflation is an issue of widespread concern whereas queueing problems receive little or no attention because of the market clearing effects of rationing by price. In a developing country the focus is again self-selecting, the acute resource constraints that limit the health care provision of such countries making the choice of the techniques to be used to improve health a fundamental and pervasive problem.

The National Health Service (NHS) was set up in 1948 to provide primary care, hospital treatment, drugs, dentistry and glasses for the British public free of any charge at the time of use and to ensure an equitable distribution of care in the UK. While some charges have since been introduced, these are of significant size only for dentistry and glasses. In general the system is still true to its universalist principles, with private practice covering only a small minority of the population. However, the NHS has frequently suffered from criticisms of its failure to meet all the potential commitments available. Waiting lists for non-urgent surgery and investigations have continued to be substantial and are a frequent source of press and political criticism. Similarly, there are equally frequent allegations of unacceptably low standards of care in British hospitals. But complaints about the system are not limited to countries with a public health service. The demand for health care is growing world-wide as aspirations and technologies change, and so any constraint on supply is bound to lead to price increases (ruled out in the UK), quality reduction, queueing or other forms of rationing. However, the method of funding does have implications for the level of provision and the impact of the supply constraint, as we discuss below.

Health economics in the UK has covered both macro-issues concerning the level of spending and its distribution and micro-issues, such as the evaluation of individual treatments. Since much of the content and implications of these micro-studies has been discussed elsewhere (see Chapter 8) and is not specific to the system of provision, we concentrate in this chapter on four macro-issues. These are (1) the method of funding and its effects on the level of provision; (2) distribution of the available resources between regions; (3) distribution of resources between individual patients and specialities; (4) distribution of resources between social classes. The concentration of distribution issues reflects the concern of researchers to examine the extent to which the

NHS has achieved the equality of service (however defined) embodied in its foundations. However, the focus on equality also has some implications for efficiency both in terms of the outputs achieved by the system and in broader social welfare terms.

Finally, the reader should note that our focus here is on the NHS. Expenditure figures take no account of private over-the-counter expenditure on patent medicines or expenditure on private health care directly or through insurance schemes. Both items are frequently included in expenditure comparisons but our purpose in the remainder of the chapter is to focus exclusively on economic aspects of the NHS only.

10.2 NHS expenditure and provision

The growth in expenditure on the National Health Service is detailed in Table 10.1. The evidence shows that expenditure has increased substantially in money terms, rather less so as a proportion of GNP.[1] Table 10.2 shows the real resources that have been provided with this expenditure. Large increases in manpower have been combined with a smaller stock of beds to treat increased numbers of in-patients and out-patients. (Approximately 5 million inpatients and 20 million outpatients per year in the 1970s compared with 3 million and 7 million respectively at the start of the NHS).

Expenditure in real terms has grown more slowly than in most Western industrial countries (Office of Health Economics, 1973), and this suggests a reluctance on the part of the government to raise expenditure to meet rising standards in a period of slow economic growth (see Section 1.5). However, slower expenditure growth does not of itself provide evidence of under-provision. Comparisons of expenditure alone are valid only if the inputs in each country are similarly priced. For example the NHS, through its position of virtual monopoly employer, has kept medical salaries (and the wages of other groups) in check. Given the high labour content of health services, lower expenditure in Britain results. By comparison with countries operating fee-for-service, where opportunities for supplier-induced demand exist, doctors in the NHS are relatively badly paid. Thus, lower expenditure per head

Table 10.1 Public Expenditure on the NHS (£ million)

	1951–2	1961–2	1971–2	1972–3	1973–4	1974–5	1975–6
Current expenditure[a]							
Hospitals	268	538	1341	1535	1774	2662	3687
General medical services	48	88	196	212	228	265	341
Dental	36	52	122	132	147	204	239
Pharmaceutical	53	78	249	285	313	440	485
Local authority services	39	81	146	167	188	—[b]	—[b]
Total current	477	875	2152	2441	2759	3793	5065
Capital expenditure	24	52	210	255	296	302	405
Total expenditure	501	927	2362	2696	3055	4095	5470
Percentage of GDP	3.6	3.8	4.5	4.5	4.4	4.9	5.4

[a] These are the major items only and hence do not sum to give the total in row (6)
[b] Taken over by central government, 1974

Sources: *Social Trends* (1970); *Annual Abstract of Statistics* (1977)

Table 10.2 Provision and Utilisation: Health Service Provision and Use per 10,000 Persons, England and Wales

	1953	1960	1970	1971	1972	1973	1974
Hospitals							
In-patient Beds	108.4	104.7	93.1	92.2	90.3	88.9	86.8
Occupied Beds (all)	96.1	89.6	76.1	75.4	73.8	70.8	69.3
Occupied Beds (psych.)	45.6	43.3	34.7	34.8	33.9	32.7	31.3
Medical and Dental staff (wte)[a]	2.4[b]	2.8[b]	4.8	5.0	5.3	5.5	5.7
Professional and technical staff (wte)[a]	3.4[b]	4.1[b]	7.2	7.6	7.9	8.3	8.2
Nursing and midwifery staff (whole time)	32.8	35.4	38.7	39.9	42.1	42.3	68.8 (whole time and part-time combined)
Nursing and midwifery staff (part-time)	6.5	9.7	20.6	22.6	23.6	24.6	
Executive Councils							
General practitioners	4.1	4.4	4.2	4.2	4.3	4.3	4.4
Prescriptions ('000s)	49.9	47.9	54.5	54.6	56.3	57.8	60.0
Dentists	2.1	2.1	2.2	2.2	2.3	2.3	2.3

[a] whole-time equivalent
[b] whole-time only

Sources: Annual Abstract of Statistics, various years

in Britain than in parts of Europe could still result in similar health service provision.

In terms of the manpower and resources provided by the NHS, levels of provision per head of population are broadly comparable with Western Europe (see Tables 10.3 and 10.4). Therefore, it cannot be concluded that the NHS has been neglected owing to public control, though we consider below the more complex interaction between provision and use which sheds further light on the appropriateness of the level of provision. Table 10.1 also provides details of the share of resources spent by each type of service in the NHS. Hospitals have dominated the picture throughout, reflecting the priority attached to interventionist medicine as opposed to primary care and community services. The relative concentration of hospital spending in acute short-stay hospitals has led to inequalities in provision which we consider further in a later section.

Table 10.3 International Comparisons: Provision of Health Manpower (per 10,000 population)

	Doctors 1970	Dentists 1970	Nurses 1969
England and Wales	12.3	2.7	31.7
Scotland	13.3	2.6	27.4
Northern Ireland	13.3	2.7	36.5
Republic of Ireland	10.7	2.1[a]	37.2[c]
Sweden	13.6	8.4	38.2
Norway	13.8	8.2	34.4
Denmark	14.4	7.0	47.2
Finland	10.2	5.7	35.5
Netherlands	12.5	2.5	44.8
Belgium	15.4[b]	1.9[ab]	10.2[d]
Luxemburg	10.6	3.1	23.2
France	13.2[a]	4.3[a]	25.8
Italy	18.1	—	6.5
West Germany	17.2	5.1	22.1

[a] estimated
[b] physicians including those practising dentistry
[c] 1971
[d] 1968

Source: Maxwell (1974)

Table 10.4 International Comparisons: Provision of Hospital Facilities per 10,000 Persons, 1969

	General hospitals		Psychiatric hospitals	
	Beds	*Admissions*	*Beds*	*Admissions*
England and Wales	40.7	1004	38.3	30.9
Scotland	48.3	975	50.2	40.5
Northern Ireland	—	—	—	—
Republic of Ireland	39.3	1200[b]	57.0	67.2
Sweden	67.1	1470	62.8	79.4
Norway	50.2	1164	21.6	18.8
Denmark	—	1381[b]	—	39.9[d]
Finland	43.0[a]	1019[b]	42.8	80.4
Netherlands	47.9	921	—	10.2[c]
Belgium	46.8[a]	931	—	27.0
Luxemburg	57.9	1084	40.7	17.5
France	45.0	712	21.9	24.6[b]
Italy	46.8	985	21.6	23.9
West Germany	65.3	1118	18.9	28.2

[a] estimated
[b] 1968
[c] 1970
[d] 1967

Source: Maxwell (1974)

10.3 The method of funding and resource provision

Although we have not accepted the argument that the NHS is markedly underfunded as compared with other European health care systems, it must be recognised that there is a mechanism by which a collective system might be expected to attract fewer resources than a market system. Buchanan (1966) has emphasised the difference between the motives of individuals as taxpayer-voters for health care and as consumers of the same. As consumers of health care individuals demand more when care is 'free' as compared with the situation where positive prices are charged. By contrast, as taxpayer-voters individuals do not pay for their own health care, as they do in a market; rather they contribute taxes to finance health care benefits to be received by others. If individuals are more concerned with the benefits they themselves receive than with those of others in society, a likely assumption, and if their preferences are reflected accurately through the ballot box, an unlikely assumption, then the supply of health care in a collective system will be curtailed to a degree that varies directly with individual selfishness. However, in reality the connection between individual taxpayer-voter preferences and the level of health care provision is tenuous. As partly indicated above, individuals do not vote directly for the size of health care budget as a separate issue; rather, they vote for prospective Members of Parliament, who are members of a small number of political parties with broad political platforms combining many 'promises' which are unlikely to include the promise of the desired level of health care provision. It seems fair to conclude that within reasonable bounds the size of the NHS budget is a government decision.

It was the intention of the founders of the welfare state in Britain in the late 1940s that it should be paid for by social insurance. Each person in full-time employment had a weekly flat rate sum deducted from his pay, and a further contribution was paid weekly, nominally by the employer. This pattern of insurance alongside general taxation persists today in a revised form, but, although popularly thought of as the main source of finance for health and welfare services and pensions, it has long since ceased to make more than a small contribution to their financing. The bulk of expenditure on the health service is drawn from general taxation, as with any other public service.

Clearly, in attempting to decide whether the level of expenditure on the NHS is 'right', given the preferences of the general public, a number of items of evidence need to be considered. Perhaps the most striking of these is the survey evidence showing the high popular esteem in which the NHS is held (see, e.g. Political and Economic Planning, 1961, and Forsyth, 1967). Such support suggests that at the very least the NHS is regarded as good value for money, (though this may reflect the misconception that social insurance contributions finance it wholly). But direct evidence on what the public wants is limited and public preferences cannot be inferred from ballot box decisions. While the main political parties differ on the extent to which they favour expansion of health services and the introduction of direct charges, the popular support for the NHS means that it is never a central election issue. Thus Conservative plans to bring in charges were contained in their election programme in 1970 yet dropped subsequently although they had a solid majority in Parliament on other issues. Similarly, proposals by the BMA (British Medical Association, 1970) to introduce voluntary and compulsory health insurance were never taken up in spite of evidence that only 30 per cent of the population favoured higher taxes to improve the NHS (see Harris and Seldon, 1971).

The alternative source of evidence concerns the operation of the NHS and its ability to provide the services asked of it by the public. The most readily available data providing an apparent index of unmet demand are the numbers of people awaiting treatment. At first glance Table 10.5 appears to support the argument that the NHS should be expanded. Almost all the major surgical departments have experienced longer queues recently than at any time in the past. But such evidence requires more than casual interpretation. In particular we need to inquire more closely into the balance between supply and demand during the past thirty years.

We have discussed in some detail earlier in this book (Chapter 4) the role of the doctor in converting a perceived medical need into a demand for health service resources. The implications of the doctor's position as supplier and effective demander are that

Table 10.5 Hospital Waiting Lists by Major Specialities per 100,000 Population at Risk, England and Wales

	1950	1960	1970	1971	1972	1973	1974
General surgery	283.0	325.6	322.7	289.8	276.5	297.0	311.2
ENT	455.2	216.5	237.7	220.6	217.2	226.2	215.4
Traumatic and orthopaedic surgery	76.7	100.6	146.4	146.4	145.0	161.4	172.0
Opthalmology	57.1	60.2	63.0	56.2	54.3	56.0	65.0
Urology	6.3	12.2	27.0	24.0	24.0	29.7	32.6
Plastic surgery	16.5	39.7	57.9	59.0	60.3	65.3	66.0
Dental surgery	3.4	14.8	31.3	31.9	32.8	38.8	44.2
Gynaecology[a]	243.2	262.8	350.3	331.5	306.6	317.5	293.1

[a] per 100,000 women

Source: Digest of Health Statistics, Health and Personal Social Security Statistics.

the two will be systematically related in accordance with his objectives. In the NHS, supply has increased owing to increased inputs of labour and other non-capital resources, permitting a higher number of cases to be treated per year with fewer hospital beds. But this has apparently no effect on waiting lists (see Feldstein, 1964, Culyer and Cullis, 1975, 1976) because of the medical response. For example, general practitioners aware of the length of waiting lists at local hospitals are unlikely to refer potential patients when the list is long yet may reduce the standard used to decide on referrals when the list is short. Since the population at large will never be wholly healthy, because of the effects of age, consumption of the 'fruits of life' and other reasons, the scope for bringing forward new patients is enormous. Indeed, the evidence of the widespread prevelance of undetected disease suggests that, if the NHS ever found itself with a shortage of patients, the introduction of screening in the community would rapidly generate additional work (see e.g. Brown, 1973). However, such evidence raises the same question as the discussion above. The definition of ill health, whether according to some standard test (in which some 'abnormal' people are statistically bound to occur regardless of how well they feel) or according to a variable criterion determined by the availability of treatment, effectively ensures that health services on whatever scale and however funded will not keep pace.

Further influences on the level of expenditure in the NHS have been the change in medical technology and its effects on public expectations. Technological change has increased the number, sophistication and cost of major and minor surgical operations. For example, in the period 1967–73 operations on the heart increased by 73 per cent, the number of heart pace-makers inserted grew five-fold and joint replacement operations more than doubled (Owen, 1976). Yet there is no evidence to suggest that underlying patterns of illness in Britain changed at such a rate during this period. Rather, the availability of treatment and its recommendation to general practitioners and the public at large create a demand for the new treatment. For example, joint replacement has become a widespread surgical technique for which long waiting lists exist. Yet before the techniques were developed the patients currently waiting were receiving palliative drugs only, but no waiting lists existed. Similarly, the extended use of drugs as a means of dealing with problems without a direct physical cause (e.g. depression) has dramatically altered the pattern of expenditure on the drugs prescribed by general practitioners even though the incidence of depression may be unchanged.

The essential difference between the NHS and systems requiring some financial payment for care by the patient is that everyone is encouraged to come forward and rationing according to an assessment of priority is inevitable. Perfect health is unattainable, but so long as it is pursued by the medical technology, waiting lists are likely to remain a persistent feature of a system without prices as a rationing device. Furthermore, since much of the technical impetus is directed against diseases such as cancer, with expensive and extensive treatment of (in many cases) limited effectiveness absorbing considerable resources, waiting lists for surgical repair of conditions such as hernia are likely to persist regardless of any increases in resources. If evidence of manifest under-provision is to be sought it should be drawn from comparisons of health states, as reflected in the imperfect indicators available, between countries similar to Britain. In this respect there is no clear evidence to suggest that Britain is suffering from a shortage of health services on the scale suggested by waiting lists since mortality in middle age and sickness absence from work in Britain, for example, are comparable with other West European countries (see Maxwell, 1974).

10.4 The regional distribution of health service resources

10.4.1 The hospital sector

Having argued that the presence of a queue and allocation according to priority are not necessarily signs of under-funding, we should not overlook one aspect of health service spending in Britain that does suggest under-provision and as a result, unequal provision. This is the hospital building programme.

In 1948 the health service took control of the voluntary and local authority hospitals that existed at that time. Since these had been constructed according to local rather than national decisions, they reflected local philanthropy and concern rather than national policy. It would have been surprising if the distribution had been uniform *per capita*. Nor was the distribution systematically related to geographic patterns of ill health, since, while more disease in an area may have called forth more local government or philanthropic action, inequalities in underlying income levels would have prevented the achievement of a desirable national pattern of hospital provision.

Detailed data on the age of hospital buildings are difficult to obtain but Owen (1976) writing after a period as Minister of State for Health, has reported that 48 per cent of British hospitals were built before 1918 compared with 16 per cent of secondary schools and 42 per cent of primary schools. Comparisons with housing are equally unflattering. Almost half of Britain's housing stock was built after 1948 but only a quarter of hospitals currently in use were built in that period. Indeed, from 1948 to 1965 major capital projects involved building only six hospitals. Since the mid-sixties this situation has altered, with seventy-one hospitals having been built up to 1975, but the slow pace of hospital development has left many towns of Britain with buildings physically and hygienically unsuitable for the practice of medicine. It has also contributed to the regional imbalance by failing to remedy the inherited inequalities between regions. The details of this inequality are provided in Table 10.6.

The timing of hospital construction should not be taken as a sign of Labour Party election fervour in 1964, since the Hospital Plan (Ministry of Health, 1962) was drawn up by the Conservative Government. However, the slow pace of growth prior to the

Table 10.6 Regional Inequality: Availability of Selected Types of Hospital Bed per 1000 Persons at Risk, England and Wales, 1973 (Regional Hospital Boards—Now Superceded)

	Acute	Geriatric[a]	Obstetric and GP maternity[b]	Psychiatric
England	3.0	8.8	2.4	3.6
Newcastle	3.3	9.2	2.6	3.6
Leeds	3.2	11.0	2.6	3.7
Sheffield	2.5	9.1	2.4	2.8
East Anglia	2.4	8.7	2.3	2.9
NW Metropolitan London	3.6	6.7	2.3	3.4
NE Metropolitan London	3.5	8.9	2.4	3.1
SE Metropolitan London	3.4	7.8	2.5	3.3
SW Metropolitan London	3.5	7.2	2.4	7.0
Oxford	2.3	9.9	2.3	2.8
South West	2.5	9.0	2.6	4.5
Birmingham	2.7	10.2	2.3	3.1
Manchester	3.1	9.2	2.5	3.1
Liverpool	4.0	9.1	2.6	3.5
Wessex	2.4	7.8	2.3	3.5
Wales	3.4	9.2	[c]	3.2

[a] per 1000 persons 65+
[b] per 1000 women 15–44
[c] Welsh statistics non-comparable

Source: Digest of Health Statistics, Health and Personal Social Security Statistics

1960s may have been influenced by the prevailing view of health and health services and broader links with macroeconomic policy. It was originally anticipated that health would improve following the institution of the NHS and that health services would naturally command fewer resources. Clearly in the 1950s adherents to such a view of health would have suggested that expansion and improvement of the hospital capital stock was unnecessary, thus saving the economy's building resources for other social overhead capital. Subsequently, the links between the NHS, public spending and macroeconomic policy suggest that the pace of hospital building will always be slow.

Keynesian macroeconomic policy requires manipulation of the level of public expenditure to secure full employment or external trade balance. Such manipulation inevitably falls on the larger items of public expenditure such as health services if only because their exclusion from such control would imply even larger variations in other items of expenditure. Furthermore, the rapid increase in medical technology has raised the cost of hospital construction, by altering standards for their facilities and equipment, to an order of magnitude of £10,000-plus per bed in acute general hospitals. Indeed, such is the cost of a new hospital that we may never again see new buildings of the standard provided in the early 1970s in Britain, because to build to the highest standard of excellence will concentrate the capital programme into relatively small areas and few beds.

It has been proposed (British Medical Association, 1977) that the NHS be separated from such direct control by governments through the setting up of various charges. This would undoubtedly have the advantage of removing macroeconomic controls from health service budgets, but such freedom is unlikely to be granted in view of the sheer size of the required modernisation budget and the undesirable consequences of charges on individuals and on resource allocation.

Finally, critics of modern health services such as Illich (1976) and McKeown (1976) have suggested that concentration on sophisticated hospital medicine is an inappropriate direction for future development. Thus, at first sight the slow pace of hospital building might appear highly desirable in that it reflects falling government norms of required beds per head of population. But given that 'technological' medicine is still practiced, slower replacement leaves some areas of Britain with fewer hospital facilities even for simple and effective surgery.

A further consequence of the unequal distribution of hospital capital has been its effects on revenue distribution. In the period 1948–70 the method of funding was essentially incremental, giving each region an amount based on the previous year's budget with adjustment for new services and for inflation of wages and prices. Thus, regions that were relatively poorly provided with hospital beds did not receive any additional revenue, beyond that pre-empted by their share of the national capital stock, with which to finance alternative services or a faster throughput of cases, and hence they were unable to compensate for their capital deficiency.

10.4.2 A new policy for equity

In 1970 a first attempt was made to allocate revenue for the funding of regional hospital services on the basis of population. While this initial attempt was in many respects unsatisfactory (see West, (1973), for a detailed discussion), it was the beginning of a new policy towards the allocation of resources for all services except general practitioners that culminated in the recent development of a detailed formula, the report of the Resource Allocation Working Party (Department of Health and Social Security, 1976a), hereafter known by its acronym RAWP.

RAWP's terms of reference, asking for recommendations with a view to 'securing . . . a pattern of distribution responsive objectively, equitably and efficiently to relative need' (DHSS, 1976b, p. 5) were set in May 1975. While neither of the present authors was privy to the underlying political pressures leading up to this commission and its 1970 forerunner, it is plausible to argue that the constraints on public spending imposed by macroeconomic policy again played a role. In a service such as health care, where quality is of pre-eminent concern, it is tempting to embark on policies that achieve equality by raising each region to the standards of the highest rather than by bringing all regions closer to the average. But such policies can succeed only in periods of growth in the total resource input. When the total is fixed, equality 'at the average' requires an allocation scheme that can be seen to be objective and justifiable.

The first step towards setting equitable capital and revenue targets is the establishment of the regional population base. Clearly an allocation of resources to each region based solely on its crude total population is equitable only if regions are, per head of population, equally in need of health services. Typically they are not, as far as can be determined from available data. The age structure of a region is one major determinant of the morbidity of its inhabitants, but a wide range of other factors such as occupations, social and ethnic grouping and environment may all have an impact on morbidity. RAWP proposed two adjustments to crude populations in order to provide a morbidity-adjusted basis for allocation. Age is taken account of by a series of weights reflecting the use of hospital services by each age–sex group. The national average number of days spent in hospital per year for each group is multiplied by the number in that group and then totalled to give regional age-adjusted population. Such a weighting scheme is open to the criticism that the old, while spending many more days in hospital than the young, consume fewer services of the more expensive acute kind when they are there. However, more refined weighting based on resource use is not yet possible because hospital costs are itemised and accounted for by department and not by patient. Thus the RAWP proposal, similar to the 1970 formula's population age adjustment, is very much a first approximation. Regional differences in morbidity owing to factors other than the age structure of the population are taken account of in the RAWP report by a further weighting of the age-adjusted population. The weights used are the standardised mortality ratios for each region. These show the number of deaths in the region as a percentage of the number that would have occurred in that region if the national average pattern of mortality in each age–sex group had occurred in the region. These ratios show as much as 13 per cent above average mortality in the Mersey region and 12 per cent below average in East Anglia (in 1971), indicating the scale of this dimension of inequality of well being.

Mortality-based adjustment is not, however, without its shortcomings. In particular, the incidence of many diseases that cause substantial illness but few or no deaths is inadequately reflected in mortality data. While this is partly overcome by the RAWP proposal that mortality data be disaggregated and rare causes of death (e.g. skin diseases) omitted, the general shortcoming that mortality reflects only one, albeit the most significant, facet of morbidity remains. A further drawback is that, since a large number of deaths occur in hospital where the patient is receiving the acute care for which the NHS is renowned, high death rates may not indicate a resource deficiency and may not be reduced by a more favourable reallocation. Rather they may draw funds and emphasis away from less critical but more readily remedied disorders. However, at present data limitations mean that regional morbidity adjustment is necessarily based on mortality figures, the only data routinely collected with sufficient detail. West (1978) has shown that the limited data available from other sources do not wholly confirm the pattern of morbidity suggested by age and mortality adjustments alone, but a more conclusive verdict must await further research.

The RAWP document is a highly detailed one and it covers a wide range of services such as out-patients and ambulances with further population weighting schemes; but the discussion above covers its main component and its main methodology. Finally, the reader should note that the dominance of population in determining the capital and revenue shares of each region (as targets to be approached gradually in order to avoid undue dislocation) is a major departure even from the earlier 1970 formula, which contained substantial elements reinforcing the unequal pattern. Not surprisingly, the cuts in spending and disappointments for some regions have made its introduction a controversial subject and a continuing subject for debate.

10.4.3 Distribution of general practitioners

The present distribution of general practitioners providing primary care in the UK has as one of its root causes the method of remuneration negotiated prior to the inception of the NHS. It was the original intention of the Ministry of Health that general practitioners would change from being free agents charging a fee-for-service to salaried employees of local government authorities. However, the general practitioners defended their autonomy vigorously and secured agreement on a method of payment that freed them from direct local government control – the capitation fee.

General practitioners (GPs) receive an annual fee for each patient on their list, i.e. all the people registered with their practice. Although there are some additional payments, the income from capitation fees, which are paid to the GP from tax revenue, form the main component of income. In principle this method of payment provides an incentive for doctors not to concentrate geographically, since to do so means sharing a limited population (and fee income) more ways. However, an unequal distribution persists for a number of regions. First, although there is some incentive to avoid clustering the incentive may be weakened by taxation. Any loss of income owing to concentration is reduced since a part of the extra income from relocation would be lost in taxation. Against this the fringe benefits of living in the less industrial areas of the UK provide compensation. This is partly reflected in regional statistics showing list sizes of around 2450 in the industrial areas of England, 2180 in the South-West and Wales and 2000 in Scotland. But these figures mask the more detailed breakdown of the distribution. Within industrial regions individual areas have substantially larger GP lists.

Some attempts have been made to reduce disparities by preventing the entry of additional GPs into an area and by introducing additional small payments for GPs in an area designated as being under-provided.[2] But these payments have had little effect, possibly because of high marginal tax rates. Also, Butler *et al.* (1973) have found that family ties and the place of training exert considerable influence on GPs choice of area. Hence a policy of establishing medical schools in under-provided regions has been pursued in order to improve the provision of GPs as a spin-off from national medical education. However, embargoes, incentives and other policies are likely to succeed only in periods of growth in the number of doctors entering general practice. When the total is static, replacement in the better provided regions is likely to absorb many of those who could be reducing the under-provision elsewhere. Such levelling-out is, therefore, less likely to occur while GPs retain their quasi-independent status.

10.5 Inequalities between patients

10.5.1 Horizontal equity

Horizontal equity of health service provision can be defined as 'equal access to care and equal resource provision for a patient with a given condition of given severity regardless of where he lives'. If such equity existed, we would expect a 'standard' patient to receive the same treatment after the same waiting time throughout the UK once the regional inequalities discussed in the previous section had been removed. However, there is ample evidence suggesting that differences in resource provision have been magnified and distorted by the way in which medicine is practised.

The principle of 'clinical freedom' concerns the freedom (and responsibility) of a doctor to choose the best treatment from those available. But medicine in practice is not the exact science of the laboratory. In the absence of controlled experiments and given the ethical problems of introducing them (not to mention the required admission by doctors that they are uncertain as to what *is* the best treatment), wide divergencies in treatment policy remain. These are particularly important in hospital since, although most cases are dealt with by general practitioners, the greatest share of expenditure is concentrated in the hospitals and the resource consequences of differences are substantial. Owen (1976) has observed that expenditure on hospitals suggests that each doctor is responsible for allocating around £100,000 of resources per annum or, if decision-making is seen as concentrated in the hands of consultants (the heads of the medical teams), £500,000 per decision-maker. Thus even at 10 per cent excess, spending by one consultant on unnecessary care involves perhaps £50,000 of resource misuse.

The assessment of the extent of divergence in treatment is complicated by the difficulty of making accurate comparisons. However, discrepancies too large to be plausibly explained by medical factors alone have been found, after adjustment for age and sex, in the treatment of a number of common conditions; e.g., Cooper (1975) has noted that the length of stay for hernia repair varies between hospitals by a factor of five and for appendectomy by a factor of six. More specific studies confirm the scale of such variations. Heasman (1964) found that, while in one hospital area four-fifths of children having operations to remove tonsils stayed in hospital for six days, half those treated in another area were discharged after one day. (For a review of further evidence, see Cooper, 1975.)

There is considerable evidence to suggest that such variations extend across general practice also, with referrals to hospital varying substantially between doctors without any apparent differences in underlying morbidity. Similarly, GPs are free to prescribe the drugs of their choice and are, as a result, bombarded by a mass of advertising from drug companies extolling the merits of their drug in spite of the enormous amount of duplication and the frequent existence of cheaper non-branded equivalents.

The discussion above brings us back to the broad issues of equality and efficiency. Not only are patients treated differently between hospitals, but such inequality also implies inefficiency.

The work load of hospitals could be cut substantially or the number of cases treated increased if length of stay were standardised for unexceptional cases.[3] But doctors have religiously guarded their clinical freedom so that any attempt to standardise would almost certainly be met by an assertion that the patient is their responsibility. Their frequent failure to demonstrate responsibility of resource use in the best interests of all present and potential patients suggests that clinical freedom will remain an issue in the future. Indeed, it is perhaps inevitable that it will, since hospital management is faced with the task of controlling overall a set of highly heterogenous production techniques given uncertain demand and a highly skilled, independent and necessarily flexible work force. Medicine is one of the few industries where the most highly educated and independent members of the work force are most directly and, for surgery, manually involved in the production process. Shop-floor autonomy becomes both an asset and a liability in such a system, and striking a balance will remain a difficult and sensitive issue. However, some steps have been taken to limit the inefficient use of resources, e.g. by notifying doctors, without criticism, of their practices compared with that of their colleagues in terms of e.g. length of stay per patient. Since ultimate responsibility will inevitably remain with the doctor, it may be that this kind of moral suasion together with the setting of broad priorities and budgets represents the most viable method of increasing the efficiency of the NHS.

10.5.2 Vertical equity

By vertical equity we mean here the extent to which individuals suffering from different disorders receive appropriately different health services. In particular we are interested in the patterns of care in different departments of the health service. As standards for comparison we focus on three areas: medicine aimed at saving life, medicine aimed at improving the quality of life, and chronic care for those with no prospect of improvement (e.g. the old, the mentally handicapped). At present the NHS still endeavours to make the best possible care available in emergencies, though it is not always able to treat all cases requiring life-saving care for long periods (e.g., renal dialysis is not currently available for all who require it). Waiting lists for non-urgent cases (some involving major surgery) have persisted for reasons already noted. But the quality of care ultimately provided is rarely criticised. It is in the care of geriatric and mentally ill patients that relatively low standards of care obtain. There have been several scandals at individual psychiatric hospitals where patients have been generally maltreated and have received virtually nothing beyond custodial care. Such scandals are symptomatic of the general problem of provision for those requiring care but for whom the possibility of cure is remote.

The extent of the inequality of provision is shown in the expenditure figures for hospitals of different types. In 1975–76 expenditure per patient day in acute hospitals was £31 compared with £12 per day in geriatric hospitals, £10 in mental illness hospitals and £9 in mental handicap hospitals. While these differences in expenditure are due partly to the greater input of technical equipment required for acute care, they also indicate the priorities implicit in present patterns of expenditure. For the emergency case care will be the best possible. For those in need of care rather than cure, provision is still frequently inadequate.

Given the limited success of high-technology medicine in saving life (see Powles, 1973) it is clear that priorities need to be rethought as proposed recently (DHSS, 1976b). Essentially it is current policy to redirect resources, albeit slowly, towards providing more care for the growing numbers of elderly people and for primary services that provide a less costly but effective method of dealing with health needs. Similarly, greater emphasis has been placed on prevention (DHSS, 1976c) as a potentially very low-cost method of avoiding future health problems, and medical care expenditure.

The Radical Statistics Group (RSG) (1976) has been highly critical of the two government papers on priorities and prevention. Their argument is derived partly from the failures of the NHS that the documents make manifest. The mental health services, for example, are a current priority. Yet such services have been stated priorities of policy in the past with little or no effect (e.g., revenue expenditure for the mentally ill fell from 12.9 per cent of the total in 1964–65 to 11.3 per cent in 1973–74). RSG have also highlighted the key role of staff in the NHS. Since staff absorb around 70 per cent of the NHS budget, any shifting of expenditure implies a shifting of staff. Yet the policy documents offer little explanation of how this is to be achieved in the face of reluctance on the part of the medical profession including nurses, etc., to practise in the less attractive specialities such as mental illness and geriatrics.

In similar vein the RSG have criticised the failure of the policy documents to emphasise the adverse health effects of industrial society and to prepare legislation and expenditure to oppose them (e.g. preventive health expenditure rising to approximately £20 million by 1979–80, measured at 1974 prices, compared with £65 million spent in advertising alcohol and tobacco alone).

The reallocation of health service resources between different areas of medicine raises fundamental issues of the importance of each dimension of medicine and its contribution to social wellbeing. These cannot be readily resolved given the limited availability of evidence on the success or otherwise of much of medical practice. But in the long run they will inevitably have to be faced, since the high cost of intervention with sophisticated technology is effectively limiting its application to only a few. Furthermore, we may need to face the further problem that preventive measures may not succeed. Smoking has fallen in the UK in recent years but not to an extent where the anti-smoking lobby can claim more than limited success. (For the period 1961–73 male smokers fell, as a percentage of the population from 59 to 49 per cent, but the 43 per cent of the female population smoking remained unchanged: (Owen, 1976.) If similar results were to follow the discovery of other links between various consumption goods and health, the prospect of a decline in the demands placed on the NHS seem dim. It will then be an urgent matter of policy for the NHS to decide how far it can retain its commitment to 'free' care for all in the face of rising costs of intervention.

10.6 Inequalities between social classes

In a system in which individuals are encouraged to present themselves for treatment free of any direct charge we might expect that, given the decisions on budgets and priorities, health care of any particular type would be allocated independent of factors such as income. Thus, while there would be differences in the illnesses presented by each social class, owing to, for example, occupational factors and levels of consumption, these should meet with a medical response based on need. However, there is now a growing body of evidence suggesting that members of socioeconomic groups 5 and 6 (semi-skilled and unskilled manual workers) fare less well in the health service than those in classes 1, 2 and 3 (professional, managerial and skilled manual/clerical).

The differential incidence of ill health in particular social classes is relatively easily demonstrated by routine statistics and individual surveys. Indeed, concern with the differential mortality in low-income groups was the spur to the development of social class mortality statistics, the first of many inquiries into deprivation in Victorian England. While the extent of inequality has unquestionably fallen since then, current data suggest that substantial differences in health remain. Thus, recent research has shown that birth weight is lower and mortality higher for babies born in lower social classes. Similarly, standardised mortality ratios are consistently higher in lower social classes (see Reid, 1977). Nor is it the case that members of higher social classes suffer from a greater incidence of some 'rich man's diseases'. Rather, the differential is less for some diseases (e.g. heart disease) than others (e.g. lung cancer and bronchitis), but it never reaches zero for any of the major causes of adult mortality.

The pattern of greater ill health for those in the lower social classes is confirmed by data relating to morbidity rather than mortality. The Office of Population Censuses and Surveys (1975) General Household Survey for the year 1972 showed that self-reported sickness of both chronic and acute (i.e. short duration restriction of activity) kinds exhibited a consistent gradient across social classes with the rate for class 6 being more than double the class 1 rate for chronic illness. A similar pattern is confirmed by studies and data on a wide range of different aspects of illness (for surveys of such data see Reid, 1977; Backett, 1977).

It is not our intention here to pursue the various causes of differential ill health. Rather we turn to the evidence on differential use of services. Clearly, the patterns of disease summarised above would lead us to expect greater use of health services by lower social classes. Rein (1969) has argued that members of lower social classes make the greatest use of health services and receive care qualitatively as good as that received by higher social classes from the NHS. This view is supported by the data from the General Household Survey mentioned above, which showed that lower social classes consulted GPs 16 per cent more and attended out-patient clinics 13 per cent more than would have been expected given the age of the individuals in the sample. Similarly, members of social class 1 used both services 5 per cent less than average.

However, there are a number of illustrations of the better access to health services made possible by factors such as the education of the higher social classes and their doctors' response to them. Backett (1977) has quoted evidence of higher referral rates to hospital by GPs for patients from higher social classes. Similarly, Cartwright and O'Brien (1976) have concluded that, not only do members of higher social classes make greater use of preventive services, but they also receive better care in some respects because of the unequal distribution of facilities and their ability to communicate with doctors more effectively.

We have so far argued that illness and use of health services are both greater in lower social classes, but as yet we have presented nothing to show how far the higher utilisation is proportional to the incidence of sickness. This is because the data on illness relate to individual conditions or states of health while utilisation data are more general. In other words, we do not know how far the use of health services by a social class is appropriate, given the incidence of disease it faces. Le Grand (1978) has attempted to allocate NHS expenditure to individual social classes by looking at data on health service contacts and incidence of disease in each class. But because of the data deficiencies, it is impossible to apportion the pattern of use to particular disease. Members of social class 6, according to General Household Survey data used by Le Grand, have on average a 67 per cent lower number of consultations with a GP when they are ill than those in social class 1. Clearly, if those who are ill but do not contact the health service are seriously ill, then the health service is failing to get to those who might benefit substantially from health care. Equally clearly, if they are trivially ill the lower number of contacts is of little importance. In the absence of better data no firm conclusion on the degree of inequality of health service resource use between social classes can be made.

10.7 Summary

The present operation of the NHS clearly presents a number of problems. Waiting lists remain, as do inequalities, in a number of dimensions of provision. While we have argued that national waiting lists are not a symptom of under-provision, inequalities in the distribution and receipt of health services are indeed an important policy problem. However, the introduction of a more explicit funding scheme for hospital regions represents one step towards a reduction in inequality. Difficulties such as vertical and social class inequality may be less susceptible to changes in resource allocation if it is the behaviour of agents in the system that generates them.

It seems doubtful that the NHS will be replaced or reduced in the immediate future, given its widespread political support. But a successful search for a system of incentives and organisational structure that will make NHS decision-makers responsive to the results of research findings and central policy decisions is a prerequisite of improved resource allocation and usage.

NOTES

1. For a recent statistical investigation into the main determinants of international differences in public spending on health care since the early 1960s see OECD (1977).
2. An area is designated as under-provided with general practitioners if, after nominally allocating 2500 people to each GP in the area, a further 2500 or more of the population remain unallocated.
3. Olowokure (1978) attempted to quantify the impact various factors had on the average length of stay among acute hospitals. Although his analysis leaves a substantial proportion of variation unexplained, the rate of in-patient operation, bed supply, status and number of medical staff, local authority welfare expenditure and the rate of out-patient attendance were all identified as significant explanatory factors.

REFERENCES

BACKETT, M. (1977) 'Health Services' Chapter 6, pp. 93–132, in Williams, F. (ed.) *Why the Poor Pay More*. London: Macmillan Press for National Consumer Council.

BRITISH MEDICAL ASSOCIATION, (1970), *Health Science Financing*, London: B.M.A.

BRITISH MEDICAL ASSOCIATION (1977) 'Evidence to the Royal Commission on the NHS,' *British Medical Journal*, Vol. 1, No. 6056 (20 January), pp. 314–16.

BROWN, R. G. S. (1973) *The Changing National Health Service*. London: Routledge & Kegan Paul.

BUCHANAN, J. M. (1966) *Inconsistencies in the National Health Service* (Occasional Paper No. 7). London: Institute of Economic Affairs.

BUTLER, J. R., BEVAN, J. M. and TAYLOR, R. C. (1973) *Family Doctors and Public Policy*. London: Routledge & Kegan Paul.

CARTWRIGHT, A. and O'BRIEN, M. (1976) 'Social Class Variations in Health Care and in the Nature of General Practitioner Consultations', pp. 77–98 in Stacey, M. (ed.) *The Sociology of the National Health Service* (Sociological Review Monograph No. 22) Keele: University Press.

COOPER, M. H. (1975) *Rationing Health Care*. London: Croom Helm.

COOPER, M. H. and CULYER, A. J. (1970) 'An Economic Analysis of some Aspects of the NHS', in British Medical Association, *Health Service Financing*. London: BMA.

CULYER, A. J. and CULLIS, J. G. (1975) 'Hospital Waiting Lists and the Supply and Demand of Inpatient Care,' *Social and Economic Administration*, Vol. 9, No. 1 (Spring), pp. 13–25.

CULYER, A. J. and CULLIS, J. G. (1976) 'Some Economics of Hospital Waiting Lists', *Journal of Social Policy*, Vol. 5, Pt 3 (July), pp. 239–64.

DEPARTMENT OF HEALTH AND SOCIAL SECURITY (1976a), *Sharing Resources for Health in England: Report of the Resource Allocation Working Party*. London: HMSO.

DEPARTMENT OF HEALTH AND SOCIAL SECURITY (1976b) *Priorities for Health and Personal Social Services in England*. London: HMSO.

DEPARTMENT OF HEALTH AND SOCIAL SECURITY (and Scottish Office, Northern Ireland Office, Welsh Office) (1976c) *Prevention and Health: Everybody's Business*. London: HMSO.

FELDSTEIN, M. S. (1964) 'Hospital Planning and the Demand for Care', *Oxford Bulletin of Economics and Statistics*, Vol. 26, No. 4 (November), pp. 361–8.

FORSYTH, G. (1967) 'Is the Health Service Doing its Job?' *New Society*, Vol. 10, No. 264 (19 October), pp. 545–50.

HARRIS, R. and SELDON, A. (1971) *Choice in Welfare* (1970: Third Report on Knowledge and Preference in Education, Health Services and Pensions). London: Institute of Economic Affairs.

HEASMAN, M. A. (1964) 'How Long in Hospital? A Study in Variation in Duration of Stay for Two Common Surgical Conditions', *Lancet*, Vol. 2, No. 7359 (12 September), pp. 539–41.

ILLICH, I. (1976) *Limits to Medicine, Medical Nemisis: The Expropriation of Health*. London: Marion Boyars; also published 1977 Harmondsworth: Penguin.

LE GRAND, J. (1978) 'The Distribution of Public Expenditure: The Case of Health Care', *Economica*, Vol. 45, No. 178 (May), pp. 125–42.

MCKEOWN, T. (1976) *The Role of Medicine: Dream, Mirage or Nemesis?* London: Nuffield Provincial Hospitals Trust.

MAXWELL, R. (1974) *Health Care: The Growing Dilemma* (a McKinsey survey report). New York: McKinsey.

MINISTRY OF HEALTH (1962) *A Hospital Plan for England and Wales*, Cmnd 1604. London: HMSO.

NOWLAN, D (1977) 'Britain's National Health Service. Part I: Limited Money, Unlimited Demand', *Canadian Medical Association Journal*, Vol. 116, No. 10 (21 May), pp. 1176–80.

OECD (1977) *Public Expenditure on Health* (Studies in Resource Allocation). Paris: OECD.

Office of Health Economics (1973) *International Health Expenditures* (OHE Information Sheet, No. 22, May). London: OHE.

Office of Population Censuses and Surveys (1975) *General Household Survey 1972.* London: HMSO.

Olowokure, T. O. (1978) 'Variations in Average Length of Stay among Acute Hospitals', *Applied Economics*, Vol. 10, No. 1 (March), pp. 1–10.

Owen, D. (1976) *In Sickness and In Health.* London: Quartet Books.

Political and Economic Planning (1961) *Family Needs and the Social Services.* London: George Allen & Unwin.

Powles, J. (1973) 'On the Limitations of Modern Medicine', *Science Medicine and Man*, Vol. 1 Part 1 pp. 1–30.

Radical Statistics Group (1976) *In Defence of the NHS.* London: Radical Statistics Group.

Reid, I. (1977) *Social Class Differences in Britain.* London: Open Books.

Rein, M. (1969) 'Social Class and the Health Service', *New Society*, Vol. 14, No. 373 (20 November), pp. 807–10.

West, P. A. (1973) 'Allocation and Equity in the Public Sector: The Hospital Revenue Allocation Formula,' *Applied Economics*, Vol. 5, No. 3 (September), pp. 153–66.

West, P. A. (1978) 'The Assessment of Regional Morbidity'. University of Sussex (mimeo).

11 Economic Aspects of a Private Health Care System: the USA

> . . . the United States faces the dilemma of a growing consensus that all people should have relatively ready access to medical care on the one hand, and on the other, growing consternation at the cost of providing such access.
>
> *R. Andersen* (1975, p. 3)

11.1 Introduction

The private system in the title of this chapter is the United States health care system, currently the focus of considerable discussion by economists, other social scientists and the man (potential patient) in the street. The particular reason for intense discussion of the American system revolves around recent and continuing proposals to set up some kind of 'National Health Insurance' scheme in response to widespread dissatisfaction with the existing system. The chapter title is misleading in referring to a private system in a sense, because America does have a considerable public sector. This notwithstanding, it has a health care system that comes much closer to the market model than the British NHS. In 1976 57.7 per cent of the total health expenditure in the United States came from private sources, though the proportion varied for different services, being as low as 45.2 per cent for hospital care compared with 74.8 per cent for physicians' services (see Table 11.2). The discussion of this chapter is centred on two main issues which are seen to be major sources of dissatisfaction within the system. The first concerns the very considerable increases in the cost of health care, especially hospital care, seen in the United States in recent years. In order to explain the mechanisms responsible for this inflation we discuss a further model of hospital behaviour in detail. While this model is similar in many respects to those of Chapter 6, it is introduced here specifically because of its direct relevance to the US hospital cost 'crisis'. The second concerns the equally important policy problem of unequal access to health care of different income and ethnic groups.

Finally, the US discussion of national health insurance is discussed in detail. However, before turning to the individual issues we outline the statistical background of the US health care system to provide a context for subsequent discussion.

11.2 US health care expenditures: the statistical background

Expenditure on health care in the United States amounted to $139.3 billion in the fiscal year July 1975 to end of June 1976 (Gibson and Smith Mueller, 1977). On a *per capita* basis this amounted to some $638 and represented a 14 per cent increase over the 1975 figure and amounted to 8.4 per cent of GNP. Comparison with previous years' data is made in Table 11.1. The relatively stable period 1971–4 reflects the effects of the economic stabilisation programme operating from August to April of those years. The most important influence on this sharply rising total in recent years has been the rise in prices (see columns (5) to (10) in Table 11.1 and Figure 11.2 below). It is noticeable that in the last two years health care prices as estimated by the Consumer Price Index (CPI) of the Bureau of Labour rose faster than the general CPI (all items), the only exception being fees for dentists.

As pointed out above, the United States has a mixed rather than a market health care system. Table 11.2 shows the size and proportion of government finance for health care. It is evident that there is an upward trend in such government finance. This is particularly true for hospital care, which comprises the largest single item of expenditure, almost 40 per cent. The $75.6 billion of consumer expenditures comprised all direct payments[1] for health

Table 11.1 US Health Expenditures and Percentage Price Increases, Selected Years 1929–76

Fiscal year	Total health expenditure: Amount (millions)	Per capita	Percent of GNP	Price increases (%): CPI all items	Medical care total	Hospital service charges	Hospital semi-private room charges	Physicians' fees	Dentists' fees
(1)	(2)	(3)	(4)	(5)	(6)	(7)	(8)	(9)	(10)
1929	$3589	$29.16	3.5						
1935	2846	22.04	4.1						
1940	3883	28.98	4.1						
1950	12,027	78.35	4.5						
1955	17,330	103.76	4.5						
1960	25,856	141.63	5.2						
1965	38,892	197.75	5.9	1.3	2.1		5.3	3.1	2.9
1966	42,109	211.56	5.8	2.2	2.9		6.1	3.9	2.9
1967	47,879	237.93	6.2	3.0	6.5		17.3	7.4	4.5
1968	53,765	264.37	6.5	3.3	6.4		15.9	6.1	5.2
1969	60,617	295.20	6.7	4.8	6.5		13.5	6.1	5.8
1970	69,201	333.57	7.2	5.9	6.4		12.8	7.2	6.8
1971	77,162	368.25	7.6	5.2	6.9		13.3	7.5	6.0
1972	86,687	409.71	7.8	3.6	4.7		9.4	5.2	5.7
1973	95,383	447.31	7.7	4.0	3.1		5.0	2.6	3.1
1974	106,321	495.01	7.8	9.0	5.7	4.8	6.0	5.0	4.4
1975	122,231	564.35	8.4	11.0	12.5	14.1	16.4	12.8	10.8
1976	139,312	637.97	8.6	7.1	10.2	13.4	15.2	11.4	7.7

Source: Gibson and Smith Mueller (1977)

Table 11.2 Health Expenditures by Major Expenditure Type and Source of Funds, Fiscal Years 1974–76

			Source of funds ($ million)											
			Private						Public					
Expenditure type	Total	Expenditure type as a % of total	Total	Private total % of total: (3) % of (1)	Consumers	Consumers as % of total: (5) % of (1)	Other	Other as % of total: (7) % of (1)	Total	Public total % of total (9) % of (1)	Federal	Federal as % of total (11) % of (1)	State and local	State and local % of total (13) % of (1)
	(1)	(2)	(3)	(4)	(5)	(6)	(7)	(8)	(9)	(10)	(11)	(12)	(13)	(14)
1974														
Total	106,321	—	64,890	61.03	59,836	56.28	4973	4.68	41,512	39.04	27,499	28.86	14,031	13.18
Hospital care	41,020	38.58	19,594	47.77	19,081	46.52	513	1.25	21,426	52.23	14,534	35.43	6893	16.80
Physicians' services	19,742	18.57	15,083	76.40	15,069	76.33	14	0.07	4659	23.60	3363	17.03	1296	6.55
1975														
Total	122,231	—	71,361	58.38	66,584	54.47	4776	3.91	50,870	41.62	34,126	27.92	16,744	13.70
Hospital care	48,224	39.45	21,690	44.98	21,146	43.85	544	1.13	26,534	55.02	18,371	38.10	8163	16.93
Physicians' services	22,925	18.76	17,217	75.10	17,202	75.04	15	0.01	5708	24.90	4170	18.19	1538	6.71
1976														
Total	139,312	—	80,492	57.78	75,622	54.28	4870	3.50	58,820	42.22	39,863	28.61	18,957	13.61
Hospital care	55,400	39.77	25,004	45.13	24,352	43.96	652	1.18	30,396	54.87	21,394	38.62	9002	16.25
Physicians' services	26,350	18.91	19,718	74.83	19,700	74.76	18	0.07	6632	25.17	4884	18.54	1748	6.63

Source: Gibson and Smith Mueller (1977)

services and supplies by individuals plus the total amount of premiums for private health insurance paid by individuals and/or employers on their behalf.

The role of government at all levels as a source of finance via public programmes has increased steadily since America's first extensive commitment to public health care programmes in 1967, the creation of Medicare and Medicaid. (The former covers the major costs incurred by the *old* under social security for hospital and physicians' services, while the latter does essentially the same

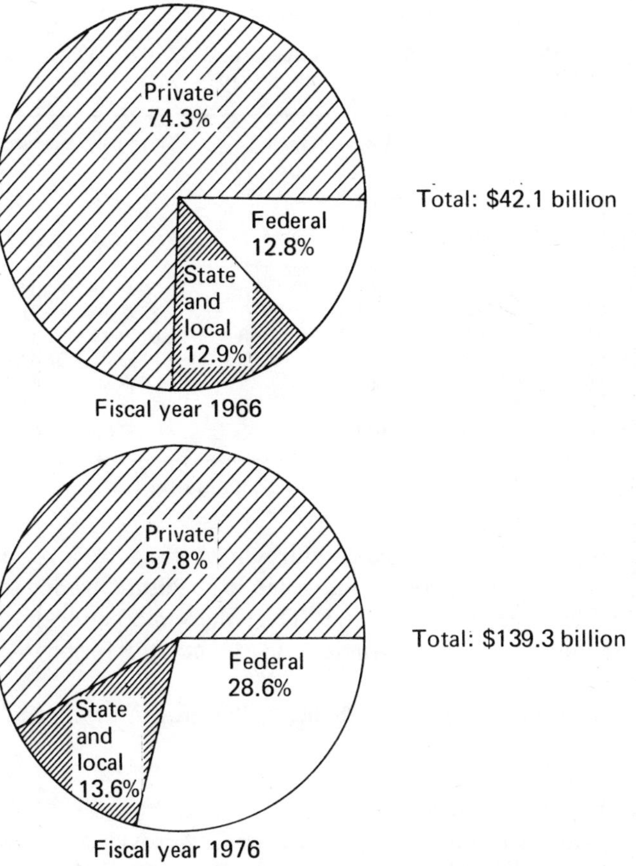

Figure 11.1 *Distribution of national health expenditures by source of funds, fiscal years 1966 and 1976.* (*Source:* Rice and Cooper, 1972; Gibson and Smith Mueller, 1977)

for the *poor*.) The decade 1966–76 has seen the government share in the total rise from just over 25 per cent to 42.22 per cent (see Figure 11.1). One of the features economists have emphasised is that the proportion of personal health services that is financed on a third-party basis has increased rapidly. (Third-party payments are those made by private health insurers or public agencies acting as insurers or providers of services.) Some relevant data are recorded in Table 11.3. It is evident that the role of third-party financing has risen from under one-third midway through this century to over two-thirds in 1976.

Table 11.3 Personal Health Care Expenditure Met by Third Parties, Selected Fiscal Years, 1949–50–1975–76

		Direct payments		Third-party payments	
Fiscal year	Total ($ million)	($ million)	as % of total: (3) as % of (2)	($ million)	as % of total: (5) as % of (2)
(1)	(2)	(3)	(4)	(5)	(6)
1949–50	10,400.4	7107.0	68.3	3293.4	31.7
1954–55	15,231.0	8922.0	59.0	6239.0	41.0
1959–60	22,727.7	12,577.0	55.3	10,152.7	44.7
1965–66	36,216.3	18,668.0	51.5	17,548.3	48.5
1969–70	58,751.5	22,929.0	39.0	35,822.0	61.0
1975–76	120,431.0	39,099.0	32.5	81,332.0	67.5

Source: Rice and Cooper (1972); Gibson and Smith Mueller (1977)

In general, US health expenditures have risen by an average of 13 per cent since 1965, the total expenditure having more than trebled since the mid-sixties. Over the same period hospital care expenditures have quadrupled and expenditures for physicians' services tripled.

The three major factors influencing the growth of expenditure are:

(*a*) price increases
(*b*) population changes
(*c*) changes in the mix of health services provided.

(a) is measured by the Consumer Price Index, and data on (b) are routinely available. However, changes in the mix of health services provided are difficult to pin down. Changes in technology in health care are rapid, and different methods of treatment become fashionable over time. Utilisation of health care is affected by insurance reducing the effective prices for care, increasing supply, etc. (see Chapter 5). Figure 11.2 indicates the influence of these factors (changes in health care systems being a catchall category) on increases in personal health care expenditures.[2]

The relative influence of the three factors has changed over time. Between 1950 and 1965 price changes accounted for 43.8 per cent of the increase, population 21 per cent and changes in the health care system 35.2 per cent. More recently, however, since the removal of economic controls in 1974, price increases have been the dominant influence. From the economist's point of view it is not sufficient to attribute the rise in costs to particular sources but rather to understand the causal mechanisms responsible. Only then can we determine whether growing health care expenditures represent an efficient use of scarce resources. This is the task of much of what follows in this chapter.

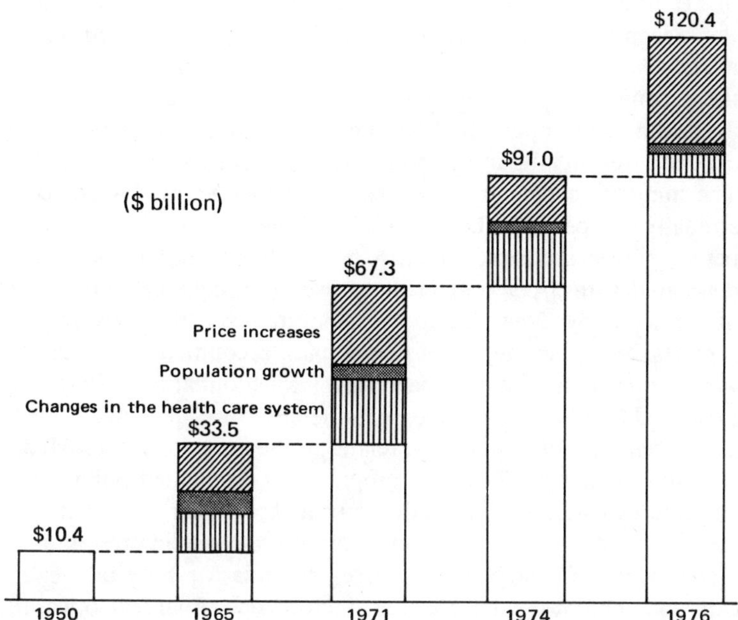

Figure 11.2 *Factors affecting increases in personal health care expenditures, selected fiscal years 1950–76.* (*Source:* Gibson and Smith Mueller, 1977)

11.3 Explaining health care cost inflation

In this section several explanations of the health care cost inflation indicated in Tables 11.1 and 11.2 are considered. As is clear from the latter, hospital care and physicians' services costs dominate total health care expenditures; hence the discussion concentrates on those elements of hospital care expenditure.

11.3.1 The price of hospital services

Between 1965 and 1976 hospital care expenditure quadrupled. Fuchs[3] (1974) has addressed himself to the question, 'why are hospital costs so high?' and has pointed out that discussion can be pursued on an *accounting* basis, i.e. breaking down hospital expenditures into their contributory components, or on a *behavioural* basis, concentrating on the actions of the main actors determining hospital expenditure – physicians and patients. The period before 1965 was characterised by relatively gentle inflation of health expenditure *per capita* compared with all services since the Second World War. After 1965 the gap widened enormously, and the cost 'crisis' dates from this time. As regards the accounting approach, it is clear that the price and quantity of health care inputs had an important influence. Since 1965 expenditures on labour and non-labour inputs have grown rapidly. The number of personnel per patient increased by 3.4 per cent annually compared with 1.7 per cent in the early sixties. Earnings per employee increased at an 8 per cent annual rate post-1965 compared with 5 per cent in the private (non-agricultural) sector of the economy. New and more elaborate medical hardware and supplies, including the use of disposables, accounted for the sharp increase in non-labour expenditures. Such inflation cannot be explained by an unusual increase in the number of patients treated.

The *behavioural* explanation relates to the introduction of Medicare and Medicaid. These two programmes dominated public programme expenditures on health care in fiscal year 1976 with 62 per cent of the total. The introduction of these public programmes made available a large new source of funds for hospital health care and the consequent demand increases were largely price-insensitive because reimbursement under the schemes was geared to the cost of providing the services.

In Table 11.3 above, the increasing importance of third-party payments was emphasised. Table 11.4 shows that third-party payments have had their greatest impact on hospital care expenditures. In 1950 direct payments accounted for 34.2 per cent of personal health care expenditure on hospital care, but the growth of private insurance in the 1950s meant that by 1965 direct payments had fallen to 18.5 per cent and the share of insurance risen from 16.5 to 41.7 per cent over the same period. After Medicare and Medicaid the private insurance share fell and government spending for hospital care rose to 54.9 per cent. Direct payments in 1976 were only 8.9 per cent. Surely it is no coincidence that this dramatic change in the arrangement of finance occurred when the 'crisis' developed! The medical decision-makers have made decisions on hospital admissions and length of stay unfettered by the third-party payers, whose role has been simply to reimburse any costs incurred by the hospital. This is not to ascribe any sinister motives to physicians and other medical care decision-makers. Their motivation seems to be to increase the quality of care in the form of additional equipment, personnel – a sort of 'Rolls Royce'-only attitude to treating each patient (see Chapter 6). Fuchs's explanation of the process draws on some of his earlier work (Fuchs, 1968), where he emphasised that the physician's approach to medical care and health is dominated by a 'technologic imperative'. This term describes the process whereby medical tradition emphasises giving the best care that is technically possible irrespective

Table 11.4 Hospital Care Expenditure by Source of Funds, Selected Fiscal Years 1950–76

	Source of funds (percentage distribution)				
		Private			
Year	Total	Direct payments	Insurance benefits	Other	Public
(1)	(2)	(3)	(4)	(5)	(6)
1950	54.3	34.2	16.5	3.6	45.7
1955	54.1	23.6	27.4	3.0	45.9
1960	58.0	18.6	36.8	2.6	42.0
1965	62.5	18.5	41.7	2.3	37.5
1970	49.2	12.3	35.5	1.4	50.8
1976	45.1	8.9	35.1	1.2	54.9

Source: Gibson and Smith Mueller (1977)

of cost considerations. The increasing role of third-party payments makes the additional treatment and care appear to be 'free lunch' for the patient, cooked by the physicians. However, at the global level such actions considerably expand the cost of hospital health care. As noted in Chapter 1, this increased expenditure does not necessarily correlate *positively* with health changes. (It is also possible that physician risk aversion due to increased negligence litigation in recent years has accentuated the process described above.)

Feldstein (1971a; 1973) has approached the analysis of inflation in US hospital costs via a detailed model of hospital behaviour similar in some respects to the Fuchs model above. Figure 11.3 provides an effective summary of the model. Quadrant (A) shows the demand curve for bed-days of hospital care at different prices. Demand is assumed to be unaffected by the quality of care but is influenced by other factors, e.g. insurance cover, which are of importance to the empirical tests. Quadrant (B) relates the price paid to the average cost of hospital care. If the hospital

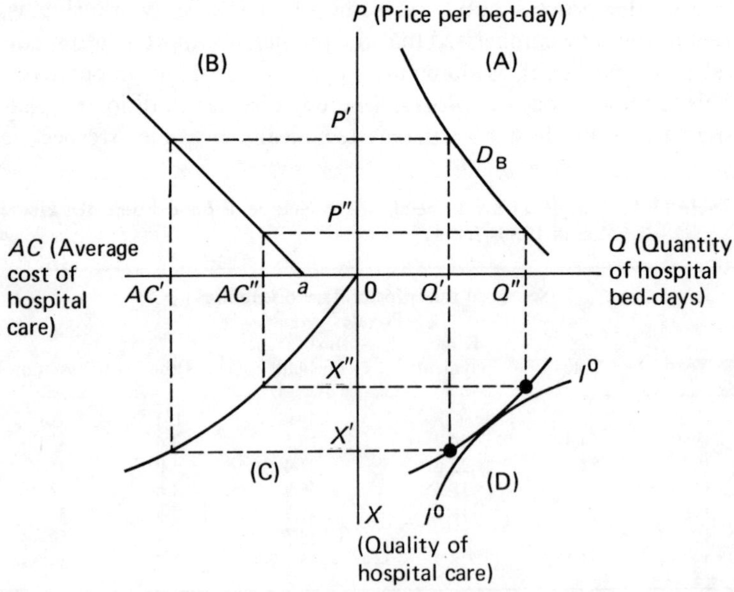

Figure 11.3 Feldstein's hospital cost inflation model

is a non-profit-making institution with some external funds to subsidise prices, then the relationship will be linear but starting from intercept *Oa*, where *Oa* is the difference between cost and price, met with external funds.

Quadrant (C) shows the hypothesised relationship between cost and the quality of care provided. Greater expenditure per day of hospital care will permit the provision of more sophisticated treatment, more comfortable facilities or more highly trained staff. Quadrant (D) then focuses on the equilibrium of the different sectors. At a given price (P' or P'') a quantity of bed-days of care (Q' or Q'') will be demanded and, in equilibrium, supplied. The prices also imply cost per day (AC' or AC'') and this determines quality (X' or X''). However, a trade-off exists between different levels of quality and the total supply of bed-days of care. If more hospital beds are provided then, because of the demand curve, the price charged will be lower. This implies a lower expenditure per day and lower quality. Thus, given the demand, cost and quality relations, we can generate the trade-off curve by finding the level of bed-supply consistent with the quantity demanded and quality provided. The task of the hospital decision-maker is to choose the combination of quality and quantity that maximises (his) utility (i.e. lies on the highest indifference curve in quadrant (D), that is I^0).

Inflation in this model is generated solely by excess demand. But this is not directly because of increases in price by hospitals in the face of queues. The hospitals are non-profit-making and so have no incentive to raise prices in order to raise revenue. However, the Feldstein model assumes that hospitals are under pressure from within to raise the quality of care. Doctors in particular may seek more sophisticated equipment in order to improve their work – Fuchs's 'technologic imperative' – and other staff will obviously exert a general push for higher wages whenever possible. Thus, when excess demand exists it provides an opportunity for these internally generated demands to be met. Prices rise as a result to the higher level consistent with the increased level of demand and the new level of quality, which again depends on the utility-maximising combination of quality and bed-supply.

An important feature of this model is that it explains the inflation of costs and the growing sophistication of hospitals without the familiar element of quality competition between hospitals that is a feature of the models presented in Chapter 6.

This makes it more consistent with the non-profit-making status of many US hospitals. Furthermore, it emphasises the role of the skilled and knowledgeable professionals, rather than the less well-informed patient, in dictating the ultimate quality of treatment.

The estimation of the various demand equations, predominantly in logarithmic form, is detailed by Feldstein. Here, our concern is with the results. These showed that demand is sensitive to (a) price, (b) the availability of hospital beds (the increase in beds presumably creating an increased awareness of health and health problems, which shifts the demand curve outwards while also lowering price), and (c) the availability of hospital specialists, increasing demand. In common with other estimated demand functions, there is a significant lag between movements in these causal variables and changes in the level of demand itself.

The empirical results clearly present a more complex picture than the earlier diagrammatic approach. Bed-supply now exerts an influence on demand. Therefore, the process by which equilibrium is achieved is no longer dependent on the hospital's decision (quadrant (D)) alone, but on the interaction between the choice of quality and bed-supply and the family of demand curves associated with each bed-stock. However, the possibility of self-generated inflation in the model (i.e. changes in bed-supply leading to an outward shift in demand, higher costs and the supply of more beds) is ruled out by the price-reducing effect of further supply, which dominates the 'pure availability' stimulus to demand.

Using the estimated demand functions, Feldstein equated demand with supply and solved the equation to find the equilibrium prices in terms of the components of demand and the supply. This price equation was then used to give an inflation equation in which the annual rate of price change is a function of the demand-influencing variables and their estimated coefficients. Thus, by regressing actual price changes on these variables, taking their coefficients as given, estimated coefficients for the impact of each demand influence on price were obtained.

The results[4] of this last stage of the regression approach show that, for 1958–67, the most important influences on hospital cost inflation (which was 91 per cent for the period 1958–67) were, in order of importance,

(a) a time trend, included to pick up the effect of improvements in technology that raise costs and prices when demand permits;
(b) the extent of insurance cover;
(c) the national consumer price index movements over the period;
(d) *per capita* real disposable income.

For the functional form which yielded a predicted rate of inflation closest to the actual rate (91 per cent), these elements contributed 48, 15, 15 and 13 per cent, totalling 91 per cent. (In addition to this however, there are several smaller influences, many of which we have mentioned already, which contribute little (5 per cent or less), have either sign and cancel each other out.)

Overall, the results fit closely with the discussion above. The time trend is accounting for the change in quality over the period and is consistent with the 'technological imperative' attributed to physicians. The extent of insurance cover brings in the role of third-party payments, while the remaining factors effectively link inflation of hospital costs to trends in other prices and incomes.

11.3.2 The price of physicians' services

In the discussion above we concentrated on hospital cost inflation, but the price inflation of physicians' services in general is also a major cause of concern in the United States. This can be linked to the operation of the three methods of paying physicians, fee-for-service, capitation, and salary. Pauly (1970) and Glaser (1970) have explored their economic implications in some detail, the major economic implications of which are reviewed below (see also Chapters 4 and 5).

Fee-for-service systems are very widespread in America. As their name suggests, the system is simply that the doctor is paid a fee for every item of service provided, e.g. general checkup, injections, X-rays, etc. Given the great ability of doctors to determine the demand for their own services, it is not surprising to find resource allocation influenced by the method of payment chosen. Fee-for-service encourages doctors to maximise productivity, i.e. maximise the number of procedures derived from given inputs; to expand the sale of units of service beyond those carried out under other forms of reimbursement, and perhaps to perform procedures unfamiliar to them in order to gain the fee for doing so (see Abel-Smith, 1976).

A capitation system is one whereby the patient pays his doctor a mutually agreed sum each time period, say a year, in return for all the care he may require in that period. Here the incentives are to minimise the costs and quantity of services (including time and trouble costs to the doctor) and thereby to maximise income – the surplus of capitation payments over expenses. Ideally the doctor would like to enroll a very large number of healthy patients at as high a capitation fee as is possible. His ability to do this varies with the degree of competition in the market. It is worth noting that preventive care is encouraged here when the costs to the doctor of preventing illness are less than those incurred should the illness develop.

The incentives associated with a salaried payment system depend on the way the salaries are to be determined. If it is by years of service alone, the motives are to minimise treatment per patient and indeed the number of patients treated. However, if the salary varies with the number of procedures carried out in some previous period, then it is in effect a fee-for-service system. The advantages of salaries are that merit can be rewarded with increases and that there is no tendency for income to fall with falling physical productivity attendant on old age, as is encountered with fee-for-service. Furthermore, salaries encourage doctors to co-operate with each other and not to see each other as financial competitors.

None of the three methods of payment for doctors is without its drawbacks. However, in view of its dominent role in American medicine, we concentrate here on fee-for-service. The typical commitment of both insurance contracts and government schemes has been to meet 'reasonable' charges *per service*. (Medicare, for example, meets 'customary' fees charged to ordinary patients.) As a result the incentives outlined in chapters 4 and 5 above are likely to lead to attempts to push up both the price and quantity of procedures provided. But it would be an over-simplification to suggest that the method of payment alone was responsible for the increase of more than 230 per cent in *per capita* expenditure on physicians' services between 1965 and 1976. On the demand side, the introduction of Medicare and Medicaid has enabled greatly increased expenditures for physicians' services on behalf of the poor and old irrespective of payment method. Other forms of third-party payments and the general income-elastic nature of health care services have also served to increase demand.

Unfortunately, increased demand has not readily been met by increased supply. For the short run at least the supply of physicians is inelastic because a physician's training is a lengthy one. Kessell (1977) has presented a supply-side explanation of the concern in America over access to medical care, in which the present problem is seen as deriving from government attempts to solve problems that are themselves a direct consequence of earlier unwarranted government intervention. The argument is that the control given to a subdivision of the American Medical Association (AMA) just before the first World War has severely curtailed physician supply. The AMA subdivision rated medical schools and made graduation from one of these schools a precondition for admission to licensure examinations. If this control over the supply of physicians had not been introduced there would be, in Kessel's view, much less concern about access to medical care today. Thus, he argued that America's health care problems stem not from any failure of the market but rather from the failure of the government to allow the market to operate in anything like a competitive manner.

To summarise, expanding private and public insurance cover have increased demand for health care by the patient (a demand-pull mechanism). The increased demand has been more than met by medical care providers, who have encouraged the provision of additional, often sophisticated and unvalidated, care (an induced demand-pull mechanism). The increased demand-pull mechanism is met by a profession artificially restricted in size by considerable entry barriers in the form of restricted places in medical schools, limited numbers of medical schools, state licensing systems, etc. (a cost-push type mechanism; for a full discussion see Kessel, 1958). The third-party payers who have met the ever-escalating bills have been powerless to stop this process, because of the dominant position of the medical profession on both sides of the market.

11.4 Equity in the provision of health care

The two standards by which equity can be judged, introduced in Chapter 10, are horizontal equity – equal treatment of equals – and vertical equity – proportionately unequal treatment of unequals. Using the approach of Chapter 10, equality and inequality of health care provision are judged by reference to the state of health of the individuals concerned. Thus Andersen (1975) has pointed out the clear implication that an equitable provision of health services ought to correlate with age, sex and marital status, as these variables indicate the likelihood of ill health. Conversely, the distribution of health care ought to be largely independent of variables such as income and race, except to the extent that racial factors are associated with patterns of income, consumption and illness.

Are the equity criteria noted above met in America? Using the economist's notion of a demand function will enable us both to highlight where inequalities might and do occur and also to give an indication of their cause. Inequalities will be measured either in terms of the presence of health care insurance policies, i.e. the *ex ante* availability of care, or *ex post*, in terms of observed quantities of care received by different individuals in society.

Assume we have a group of individuals who have a given health problem, as diagnosed by a doctor, such that on equity grounds they should receive identical treatments. What factors will lead us to observe unequal consumption of health care? The influence of the factors listed are illustrated in some cases by empirical studies that have the factor under consideration as an explanatory variable.

A knowledge of consumer theory and the earlier discussion of Chapters 4 and 5 would suggest that the following factors will influence the individual's decision to seek insurance and/or health care:

(a) the price of health care;
(b) income;
(c) other prices;
(d) tastes;
(e) information and education.

Of these, (a) price and (b) income are of obvious importance. Price effects of insurance cover have been noted earlier. Also of importance are factors such as ease of access, which affect the time-price of care that individuals face (see Section 5.3.3 above). Thus, Simon and Smith (1973) found a reduction in visits to a university health service when it moved off-campus. Income is equally central to any analysis of health care demand in the United States. Sorkin (1975) reported that in 1970 only 36 per cent of those earning less than $3000 per annum had health insurance compared with over 90 per cent coverage for those earning $10,000 or more. Of course, these discrepancies are now offset to a degree by Medicare and Medicaid, as found by Wilson and White (1977).

As for (c), other prices, a variety of substitutes and complements for health care exist. Jogging is perhaps the most noticeable attempt at a substitute, but patent remedies are still of major importance in expenditure terms, as are books on self-help. However, wider use may indicate not the search for an alternative but increased concern with health and health care. Thus, any price changes for apparent substitutes might not have the anticipated effect; e.g. if jogging acts as a form of screening.

Factor (d) – tastes – might appear a curious item to include in a book about health care. But the differences in the cultural and social environment across America, aside from links with income, can explain substantial differences in health care consumption (see Li *et al.* (1972) on the low utilisation of health services by Boston's Chinese community). Similarly, tastes for other goods may affect the incidence of ill health and the demand for health care.

Differences in information and education, factor (e) above, also explain inequalities in health care receipts. Information on the availability of health care, and the consequences of seeking or not seeking it, are likely to be very different for different individuals or groups of individuals in society. Generally speaking, it is argued that the wealthy are in a much better position to acquire information and contacts, not least because acquiring information is costly. Further, we emphasised in Chapter 2 that people are unlikely to have accurate information on the quality or price of care. As a result people operate on 'guesstimates', and those who anticipate a high price seek relatively little care compared with those who anticipate a low price for any *given* health disorder.

At the general level, then, these are the factors that influence the demand for and receipt of health care and thus help explain its inequality of distribution. It must be emphasised that, although for the sake of clarity above the demand-influencing factors have been analysed and illustrated one at a time, there is obviously very considerable inter-correlation between the factors. For example, low-income individuals probably have little information and face more cultural and social barriers to obtaining care. However, listing the various factors serves to emphasise that establishing equality in the provision of health care is likely to be much more complicated than simply transferring purchasing power to groups adjudged to be receiving too little care.

Aday and Andersen (1975) have developed indicators of access to health care that are divided into two groups, process indicators and outcome indicators. Process indicators refer to characteristics of the delivery systems or characteristics of the population at risk that affect people's utilisation of and satisfaction with care. The process indicators they have reported are: regular source of care, travel time to care, appointment or walk-in visit, appointment waiting time and office waiting time. The results indicated that: (a) older adults, fifty-five to sixty-four years of age, and the elderly must often travel more than an hour to reach care; (b) non-whites less often have a regular source of care than do whites; (c) residents of the inner-city and rural farm-dwellers are the most disadvantaged with respect to having a regular source of care that is conveniently available to them; (d) people below the poverty level are most likely to have no regular source of care, to have to travel more than thirty minutes to obtain services, to have walk-in visits and to have to wait more than thirty minutes in the doctor's office.

Outcome indicators include both objective and subjective descriptions of the population's entry to and passage through the system, i.e. utilisation and satisfaction indices, respectively. Four main indicators were reported: (a) conventional utilisation measures (percentage seeing a physician, mean number of physician visits); (b) measures of care use relative to need for services; (c) continuity of care indices; and (d) satisfaction with care indicators. Process indicators identified non-whites, rural farm and inner-city residents, the poor and those who used clinics as their regular source of care to have less access to the health care system. Outcome indicators drew much the same picture. For example, compared with the non-poor the poor were less likely to contact a physician. Although the overall use of services was similar for the poor and non-poor, it was the former group who used fewer services relative to their need. Also, the poor suffered more fragmented and less continuous care and not unexpectedly were more dissatisfied, overall, with the out-of-pocket costs and the inconvenience of health care services.

Andersen (1975), using data on 3880 families comprising 11,822 individuals, has attempted to analyse the overall equity of health service distribution. An equitable distribution of health services was defined as 'one in which illness (as defined by the patient and his family or by health care professionals) is the major determinant of the distribution' (Andersen, 1975, p. 10). The analyses suggested that, although hospital services were distributed equitably (i.e. admission by demographic and need variables), length of stay was affected by non-health status variables (e.g. social structure). Physician services were also distributed fairly equitably. However, there was evidence that 'not having a regular physician' was an inhibiting factor to making visits. Dental care was the largest source of inequity, with social structure and income being important factors in dentist visits. The study was especially concerned with the care received by the elderly, non-whites, low-income groups and inner-city and rural residents. The analysis here involved comparing health care utilisation of the subgroups with the remainder of the population. Unadjusted estimates showed that utilisation varied in the subgroups irrespective of the particular characteristics of the group compared with the remainder of the population. Adjusted estimates of utilisation were then made indicating utilisation patterns for the subgroups if the groups had the same characteristics as the whole population for each age group, e.g. marital status, ethnicity, family income, etc. This process isolated unexplained equity or excess. The major findings here were that: (a) the inner-city and rural subgroups appeared to face inequality as regards hospital admission; (b) non-whites faced inequalities in seeing a physician that were largely attributable to a lack of regular source of care; (c) dental services were inequitably distributed with minorities, rural farm dwellers and low-income individuals receiving too little treatment, partly because of financial barriers and partly because of low education and social class factors. The group most consistently experiencing inequality as regards hospital admission and doctor and dentist visits was the rural farm population.

The evidence presented here makes it clear that equity in the provision of health care is a complex notion requiring further research. However, it seems reasonable to conclude that some Americans, especially the members of the poor minority groups, do not receive or have potential command over an 'equitable' share of the nation's health care resources. This, combined with the health care cost inflation problem discussed in Section 11.3 above, has not surprisingly led to proposals for reform of America's health care system.

11.5 Proposals for reform

Economic policy proposals can usually be subdivided into three groups. Market-perfecting or improving policies are concerned with identifying those aspects of the current situation that prevent the market from operating properly and removing them or offsetting their effects. This approach involves minimum intervention by government and maximum reliance on the market and the individual utility-maximising calculus. At the opposite end of the spectrum are policies of complete government provision which are based on arguments of general or specific market failure. Between the two are policy options which attempt to draw on the advantages of both private and public provision.

Proposals for reform of the American health care system can be categorised under three heads. One pressure group, the 'market-improvers', favour a return to a largely unbridled market which they claim America has never had. 'Eclectics' and 'market-displacers' both want some form of national health insurance (NHI), but whereas the 'eclectics' want a minimum type insurance scheme the 'market-displacers' want an almost exclusive government scheme providing all health services.

11.5.1 'Market improving' policy

Havighurst (1977) has denied the need for extensive federal government intervention in controlling health care costs, by arguing that the private sector should be given a chance to put its own house in order. His thesis is that, once third-party payment patterns were established with relatively complete coverage and without cost controls initiated by insurers in the patient's interest, the spiral was set in motion. Cost increases facilitated by insurance necessitate the purchase of further insurance, thereby stimulating further cost increases and insurance cover expansion (c.f. Feldstein, 1971a).

The argument is essentially double-edged, explaining why the market has failed in the past and why in the future the market solution has much to offer. The failure of the market in the past to ensure appropriate insurance coverage and impose adequate cost controls is alleged by Havighurst to stem from two sources. First and more important is the control over the design and implementation of financing programmes by the medical care providers. It was only when hospitals and doctors themselves came to sponsor and control the practices of third-party payment schemes (Blue Cross and Blue Shield) that they became acceptable. Hence the plans developed were ones that ensured that the providers could easily collect their payments. This encouraged excessive shallow[5] 'first-dollar' coverage and insufficient coverage against low-risk and high potential cost ailments.[6] It is the latter that mean financial ruin if they strike. Commercial insurers were excluded from a role in controlling and supplying health care by the power of the medical profession, and hence schemes that involved physicians justifying their expenditure of insurers' funds were outlawed. In general, the cost-controlling efforts that insurers attempted were thwarted by the medical profession, who argued they were protecting the 'doctor – patient' relationship from damage by people who were not their peers and therefore not to be approved of.

Apart from the large measure of medical self-interest to be found in existing institutions Havighurst has drawn attention to a second artificial barrier to a more competitive (cost-conscious and consumer-orientated) situation, namely, the tax treatment of insurance premiums for health care costs. Here the problem is that tax allowances encourage employees and employers to buy group insurance with low deductibles, i.e. covering the cost of purely routine procedures (high probability, low potential cost). This is argued to be 'irrational' (see Fuchs, 1976) because for any given potential loss it is the unpredictable (low-probability) events for which the value of the service of insurance (to risk-averse individuals) exceeds the necessary 'loading' to allow for administrative costs etc.

Income tax produces this outcome by distorting the choice between monetary and non-monetary forms of income. Employers seeking to give an employee a given rise in income must include in the rise the additional tax due on the rise and hence must increase the total cost of the rise beyond its actual value to the individual. If instead the employer gives the worker a health insurance policy valued at the size of the net of tax rise, this will enable the employee to reduce personal expenditure on health care and hence he has received a non-taxable increase in income. In general, a fringe benefit is not as attractive a proposition as cash, so its value may well need to be above the after-tax value of the cash rise to be acceptable. But as long as the value of the fringe benefit required for equivalence is below the pre-tax value of a cash rise, there may well be a gain to be made. Whether there is or not will depend on the size of the transaction costs incurred by the employer in administering the health care insurance scheme. It is clear that the higher the marginal tax rate paid by the employee the more attractive fringe benefits become. This tax avoidance mechanism has, it is argued, resulted in insurance coverage of health care expenditures that would otherwise have been met 'out of pocket'. The process is reinforced by employee health care insurance purchases being tax deductible. This results in patients seeking and doctors providing care that would otherwise have seemed not worthwhile and makes further inroads into the area where the normal market cost constraints operate. The suggested reform to offset the effects of this distortion is a limited tax credit against employees' taxes for employer- and employee-paid health care insurance premiums.

The implication of this analysis is that the market has been handicapped and rendered ineffectual rather than being inherently so. The sort of cost control reforms Havighurst has proposed involves reducing insurance coverage and increasing the area of market-disciplined decisions. One example is the provision of 'major-risk' insurance. The proposed plan would have a high deductible and would maximise the role of the market, coverage beginning only when serious financial trouble was consequent on ill health. Insurers could also strengthen the bargaining position of consumers by negotiating fees and charges in advance on their behalf. Moreover, insurers may sponsor more tightly organised provider groups as a way of ensuring effective cost controls, economies of scale, quality assurance, etc. In short, there is a range of possibilities for the development and refinement of cost control strategies that would arise in a competitive health care market.

Kessel's (1977) contribution briefly summarised above is similarly a market-perfecting approach with its emphasis on the AMA's supply-restricting activities. Thus, both demand and supply could be subjected to market improvement.

11.5.2 'Eclectic' and 'market-displacing' policies

The bulk of recent policy proposals favour some form of NHI rather than the market as the solution to America's health care problems. Fuchs (1974) has provided a very perceptive view of the main issues, and it is his discussion that in part underlies this section. These are introduced below as key questions that need to be answered when framing a NHI proposal.

(*i*) *Who should be covered by NHI*? The essential issue here is 'universalism' versus 'selectivism'. Should the NHI scheme cover the whole of the population or just those who, because of lack of income or some other characteristic, find themselves excluded from health care in the current system? The case for universalism has several arguments in its arsenal. First, viewing health care as a fundamental right implies a policy proposal that relates to all, irrespective of income or other characteristics. Second, making a NHI scheme and hence the receipt of health care contingent on some sort of means test often results in low-income families facing very high 'implicit' marginal tax rates. As their income increases, not only do they pay the ruling 'explicit' marginal tax rate but they lose some means-tested benefits, which makes their share of the marginal dollar very low (and in extreme circumstances negative). Third, there is the point emphasised by Meade (1975) that, in a selective scheme, private health care insurance would probably have to be made compulsory for those outside NHI since society is unlikely to leave untreated those who become ill but lack both insurance and the means to pay unexpectedly large medical bills. However, if the improvident are treated 'free', the principle of exclusion is violated, which, from the discussion of public goods, we know encourages 'free-riders'. Fourth, it is argued that schemes designed for the poor alone quickly become 'second-class', failing to meet standards that would be insisted on by the higher-income groups. Furthermore, high-income groups form a much more successful pressure group in lobbying government because they can afford to acquire information and make party contributions, and include political leaders, so their inclusion in a NHI scheme would tend to guarantee a high standard of service.

Additionally, several points can be drawn from Britain's 'welfare state', where there have been problems in effectively providing the poor with means-tested benefits e.g. because of those who will not subject themselves to a means test, or are unaware that they are in the particular category eligible for some benefit. Furthermore, establishing eligibility is a resource-using procedure involving a large bureaucracy and time and trouble costs to the claimant that are avoided in a universalist system.

The 'eclectics' and 'market-improvers', however, might counter that a selective approach is better. The average family pays for its health care under any system so why not leave them in the market and deal with special cases ie. the poor, medically indigent etc. as the special cases they are. They see no advantage in further increasing the size of the public sector and additionally burdening the federal fiscal system. Also, the non-universalists can argue that by including only the special cases in NHI a scheme geared to their 'needs' in particular can be designed and suitably funded.

(*ii*) *What should be covered by NHI*? Here the debate revolves around whether first-dollar 'shallow' coverage of health care costs (i.e. fixed indemnity insurance with no deductible) should be included in the scheme or only major health care expenditures, the so-called 'catastrophic' costs. Some of the relevant arguments here have been mentioned above in this chapter and in Chapter 3. The main argument for 'catastrophic' coverage only derives from a concern to minimise the welfare loss associated with insurance schemes. As described in Chapter 3, the welfare loss occurs because the effect of being 'insured' against the costs of health care expenditures is generally to increase such expenditure beyond the efficient quantity.[7] Thus, while catastrophic cover must remain if the NHI system is to have the desired effect, withdrawal of the shallow coverage would remove the trivial use of services 'free' to the consumer but costly for society.

A further undesirable consequence arises if Feldstein's (1971a) hospital cost inflation model is recalled. In that model demand or willingness to pay determined costs incurred at each level of bed provision. Feldstein (1970) identified a similar effect on physician fees, with increased insurance cover resulting in increased fees (the elasticity of physician fees with respect to increased insurance cover was estimated at 0.36 per cent). Hence Feldstein's (1971b) advocacy of a high deductible 'catastrophic' cost NHI scheme and his calculation suggesting that the net gains from *decreasing* insurance by raising the average co-insurance rate from 0.33 to 0.50 or 0.67 would be of the order of $4 billion per annum. Feldstein (1973) established the latter result by estimating the gross gain from reducing health care price distortion resulting from the 'insurance' and 'cost inflation' effects outlined above and then subtracting an estimate of the welfare loss because of the increased risk borne by the family.

However, a case can be made against catastrophic coverage only, and for 'shallow coverage'. Where the latter involves widespread risk-pooling, the administrative costs of identifying who had what care are avoided and there is a gain (that Titmuss would approve of) to the non-individualist who gains from the group feeling and altruistic motives fostered by a sharing scheme. Major risk coverage only will tend to discourage health care being sought early in the development of ill health and may frustrate preventive medicine. Administration costs are likely to be substantial in a system where individuals must keep records to see if the deductible per time period is exceeded, and bureaucrats must check on cheats. Further complications arise if the deductible varies as Feldstein suggested with income and family circumstances. Moreover, once the deductible is exceeded it does not serve as a check on the quantity of care demanded by seriously ill patients, or by their doctors on their behalf, and so excessive consumption of services beyond the optimal level may still occur.

(*iii*) *How should NHI be financed and hence who should pay for it*? There are only two main contenders as the sources of finance. A payroll tax could be introduced to cover the expenses of NHI with the revenue raised going into a trust fund. Alternatively, NHI could be financed, as with Britain's NHS, from general taxation. For the United States this would mean the lion's share of the funds coming from income and corporation income taxes.

Financing NHI by a payroll tax would be the less redistributive of the above proposals. It is generally argued that the supply of labour is inelastic, so that any tax will be paid by labour as the increased price of labour reduces the demand and lowers the wage rate.

The proceeds of the tax could be paid into a trust fund and there would then be a close relation between taxes and expenditures on health care. This approach is more acceptable in buoyant economic conditions when income, employment and hence funds are also high. In periods of slump the funds will tend also to slump. However, rather than pay the proceeds of the payroll tax into a trust fund, the revenue could be placed in the general fund and expenditures on health care determined by the general budgetary processes, as with the income/corporation tax financing option. Finally, it has been noted by Fuchs (1974) and Klarman (1977) that the majority of families will pay the same under any health insurance plan but this is the case only if undesirable supply effects are prevented.

(*iv*) *How should NHI be administered*? There are two polar possibilities. The 'eclectics' and the 'market-improvers', certainly the latter, would prefer universal health insurance coverage to be achieved by compelling individuals to buy policies from private insurance companies. The federal government would have only a 'walk-on' part, involving the setting of minimum standards and ensuring that low-income and disadvantaged groups can meet their premiums. On the other hand, market-displacers have argued that 'massive national experience shows that the insurance industry adds billions of dollars in costs and distorts sensible patterns of service and expenditure, while contributing little in administration and even less in quality and cost control' (Falk, 1977, pp. 181–2). Hence even a residual role as claims-taker or fiscal intermediary for the private insurer is denied them on the grounds that the public sector can do at least as well. Arguments in favour of the single government-administered scheme include the greater control over national health care expenditure[8] afforded by a monopoly. Against this it is argued that monopoly is undesirable in either the public or private sector so that some degree of competition in administration should be encouraged.

(*v*) *How should health care under NHI be delivered*? The question here is whether the structure of the health care system needs major or only minor restructuring. Those who want organisational change see any adjustment in financial arrangements as useless without accompanying structural changes. Falk has been particularly emphatic: 'Any program with reasonable promise of success must achieve *both* cost controls *and* system improvements since neither one can be effected without the other' (Falk, 1977, p. 176; emphasis in the original). By 'system improvements' Falk had in mind a wide range of weaknesses and deficiencies. These extend from solo practice,[9] fee-for-service payments, excessive surgery and in-patient treatment to geographical maldistributions and professional control of price and expenditure levels. The prescribed alternative is a health system for all rather than the existing separate systems for rich and poor.

A popular form of health care delivery system which some argue should be used more extensively in a reformed health care system is the health maintenance organisation (HMO). HMOs are types of group practice organisations that *provide* and *assure* the member's health care for a fixed prepaid capitation fee. HMOs are popular with many commentators because of the incentive for the organisation to be cost-conscious and to maximise productivity in resource use. HMOs cover the whole range of health care services and thus avoid the externality problems that arise when the system of health care provision is fragmented into small, largely independent production units. McClure (1976) has pointed out that these externalities arise because costs and cost-saving do not accrue to the provider who creates them. When the hospital and physician are independent units, the costs of the former are not borne by the latter when a patient is recommended for in-patient treatment. The general practitioner who successfully treats an illness in its early stages receives only fees for the treatment given and no reward for the large resource savings made as a consequence of expensive in-patient treatment no longer being necessary. Pre-payment and the guarantee of health care should bad health occur encourage the efficient use of preventive medicine in HMOs. Evidence presented by McClure (1976) shows that HMOs produce comparable health results with fewer specialists and more primary physicians than the US average and do so with cost savings between 10 and 30 per cent below traditional providers. But this evidence has a double edge. The sensitive nature of medical care and the emphasis on quality (noted throughout the book) leave HMOs open to a charge of skimping on the grounds that they do not provide sufficient in-patient resources.

11.6 Summary

In this chapter the problems of health care cost inflation and equity in the US health care system have been examined. As regards the former, both demand and supply side issues were argued to have played a role. Equity was essentially viewed as being the concern to increase access to health care by the poor and minority groups and was seen to be a complex problem which would not be remedied by income transfers alone. Reform proposals designed to deal with these problems were divided into 'market-improving', 'market-displacing' and 'eclectic' options. It must be remembered that all resource use involves an opportunity cost, and extending the use of health care by the poor is no exception. Although health care is 'obviously a good thing', it is worth recalling that commentators (see Chapter 1) have observed that there is not a great deal of evidence that greater health care at the margin increases the general health status of the population. It seems likely that health status differences are either inherited or produced by life-styles and general environmental factors, and as a consequence altering these factors is perhaps a more appropriate way of altering the health status of the population at large. However, for policy purposes a distinction must be drawn between variables that can be relatively easily altered and hence used as policy weapons and those that cannot be altered readily and must, for the short run at least, be considered as parametric. In the short run, life-style and environmental factors would fall into the latter category, perhaps partly explaining the interest in the provision of health care. Furthermore, there is evidence that higher educational groups enjoy better health. If increasing the other main human resource investment – education – is an effective way to improve health status, the rationale of attempts via NHI and other reforms to increase health status by expanding the use of health care, especially by the poor, must remain, to some extent, in doubt.

NOTES

1. Direct payments are those payments made 'directly' and not through third parties such as government and private health insurance, philanthropy, etc.
2. Personal health care expenditure comprises the portion of total national health care expense that represents health supplies and services received directly by individuals.
3. Note that Fuch's book was published in 1974, so that his 'model' and discussion relate to data available only up until the early seventies. However, where relevant, some recent statistics have been added.
4. In view of the several functional forms fitted by Feldstein, these results should be regarded as illustrative rather than conclusive.
5. Munch (1976) denies that individuals have a propensity to buy shallow insurance cover, arguing that the prediction that the extent of insurance cover purchased by risk-adverse individuals will be positively related to the mean and variance of the distribution of expected losses is borne out in practice. According to Munch, data from a 1970 national survey of medical expenditures show that, for persons with annual medical care expenses below \$150, only 7 per cent was paid by insurance, and the percentage rises monotonically to 76 per cent for annual expenses above \$1500. Similarly, insurance covers a greater proportion of hospital expenses than for physician office visits, where the average total expenses are lower. The percentage of variability (measured by the standard deviation of total expense) removed by insurance is greater for hospital expenses (59 per cent) than for physician office visits (42 per cent). For book-length treatments of the American health care system see Davis (1975) and Krizay and Wilson (1974).
6. Encouraging shallow coverage is thought undesirable because all insurance policies are 'loaded' by administrative costs rather than being fair (in the sense outlined in Chapter 3), so that for risk-adverse individuals it should be worth paying the 'loaded' premium for unpredictable large losses rather than relatively certain small expenses. This conclusion is established rigorously in Lees and Rice (1965).
7. This can occur because individuals are insured in a strict sense (the situation in which ignoring administrative and other costs they have paid the fair premium $F = P(NC)$ discussed in Chapter 3) or are in a risk-pooling scheme where an individual pays a share (equal or otherwise) of the total cost of health care in any period determined by the overall use of health care services provided in that period for those in the pooling scheme, eg. the NHS.

8. Recall and contrast Newhouse's thesis (1977) discussed in Chapter 1, that all countries manage to keep their national health care expenditures in line with their resources (GNP).
9. Solo practice is disliked because, as compared with group-type practices, it under-utilises capital and human inputs as well as providing little scope for productivity increases consequent on specialisation.

REFERENCES

ABEL-SMITH, B. (1976) *Value for Money in Health Services.* London: Heinemann.

ADAY, L. A. and ANDERSEN, R. (1975) *Access to Medical Care.* Ann Arbor, Michigan: Health Administration Press.

ANDERSEN, R. (1975) 'Introduction and Health Service Distribution and Equity', Chapters 1 and 2, pp. 2–32, in Andersen, R., Kravits, J. and Anderson, O. W. (eds) *Equity in Health Services: Empirical Analyses in Social Policy.* Cambridge, Massachusetts: Ballinger.

DAVIS, K. (1975) *National Health Insurance: Benefits, Costs and Consequences.* Washington, DC: Brookings Institution.

FALK, I. S. (1977) 'Proposals for National Health Insurance in the USA: Origins and Evolution and Some Perceptions for the Future', *Milbank Memorial Fund Quarterly*, 'Health and Society', Vol. 55, No. 2 (Spring), pp. 161–92.

FELDSTEIN, M. S. (1970) 'The Rising Price of Physicians' Services', *Review of Economics and Statistics*, Vol. 52, No. 2 (May), pp. 121–33.

FELDSTEIN, M. S. (1971a) 'Hospital Cost Inflation: A Study of Non-profit Dynamics', *American Economic Review*, Vol. 61, No. 5 (December), pp. 853–72.

FELDSTEIN, M. S. (1971b) 'A New Approach to National Health Insurance', *Public Interest*, Vol. 23 (Spring), pp. 93–105.

FELDSTEIN, M. S. (1973) 'The Welfare Loss of Excess Health Insurance', *Journal of Political Economy*, Vol. 81, No. 2(1) (March/April), pp. 251–80.

FUCHS, V. R. (1968) 'The Growing Demand for Medical Care', *New England Journal of Medicine*, Vol. 279, No. 4 (25 July), pp. 190–5; reprinted as Chapter 4 pp. 61–8 in Fuchs, V. R. (ed.) (1972) *Essays in the Economics of Health and Medical Care.* New York and London: Columbia University Press for National Bureau of Economic Research.

FUCHS, V. R. (1974) *Who Shall live? Health, Economics and Social Choice.* New York: Basic Books.

FUCHS, V. R. (1976) 'From Bismarck to Woodcock: The "Irrational" Pursuit of National Health Insurance', *Journal of Law and Economics*, Vol. 19, No. 2 (August), pp. 347–59.

GIBSON, R. M. and SMITH MUELLER, M. (1977) 'National Health Expenditures, Fiscal Year 1976', *Social Security Bulletin*, Vol. 40, No. 4 (April), pp. 3–22.

GLASER, W. A. (1970) *Paying the Doctor – Systems of Renumeration and their Effects.* Baltimore and London: Johns Hopkins.

HAVIGHURST, C. C. (1977) 'Controlling Health Care Costs – Strengthening the Private Sector's Hand', *Journal of Health Politics, Policy and Law,* Vol. 1, No. 4 (Winter). pp. 471–98; reprinted as Reprint No. 68 by the American Enterprise Institute for Public Policy Research.

KESSEL, R. A. (1958) 'Price Discrimination in Medicine', *Journal of Law and Economics*, Vol. 1, No. 2 (October), pp. 20–53.

KESSEL, R. A. (1977) 'Ethical and Economic Aspects of Governmental Intervention in the Medical Care Market', in Dworkin, G., Bermant, G. and Brown, P. G. (eds) *Markets and Morals*. Washington DC: Hemisphere Publishing Corp.; reprinted as Reprint No. 67 by the American Enterprise Institute for Public Policy Research.

KLARMAN, H. E. (1977) 'The Financing of Health Care', *Daedalus* (Proceedings of the American Academy of Arts and Sciences), Vol. 106, No. 1 (Winter), pp. 215–33.

KRIZAY, J. and WILSON, A. (1974) *The Patient as Consumer – Health Care Financing in the United States* (a Twentieth Century Fund Report). Lexington, Massachusetts: D. C. Heath and Co.

LEES, D. S. and RICE, R. G. (1965) 'Uncertainty and the Welfare Economics of Medical Care: Comment', *American Economic Review*, Vol. 55, No. 1 (March), pp. 140–54.

LI, F. P., SCHLIEF, N. Y., CHANG, C. J. and GAW, A. C. (1972) 'Health Care for the Chinese Community in Boston', *American Journal of Public Health*, Vol. 62, No. 4 (April), pp. 536–9.

MCCLURE, W. (1976) 'The Medical Care System under National Health Insurance: Four Models', *Journal of Health Politics, Policy and Law*, Vol. 1, No. 1 pp. 22–68.

MEADE, J. E. (1975) *The Intelligent Radical's Guide to Economic Policy – The Mixed Economy*. London: George Allen & Unwin.

MUNCH, P. (1976) 'From Bismarck to Woodcock: the "Irrational" Pursuit of National Health Insurance: Comment', *Journal of Law and Economics*, Vol. 19, No. 2 (August), pp. 365–9.

NEWHOUSE, J. P. (1977) 'Medical Care Expenditure: A Gross National Survey', *Journal of Human Resources*, Vol. 12, No. 1 (Winter), pp. 115–25.

PAULY, M. V. (1970) 'Efficiency, Incentives and Reimbursement of Health Care', *Inquiry*, Vol. 8, No. 1 (March), pp. 114–31.

RICE, D. P. and COOPER, B. S. (1972) 'National Health Expenditures, 1929–71', *Social Security Bulletin*, Vol. 35, No. 1 (January), pp. 3–18.

SIMON, J. L. and SMITH, D. B. (1973) 'Change in Location of a Student Health Service: A Quasi-experimental Evaluation of the Effects of Distance on Utilisation', *Medical Care*, Vol. 11, No. 1 (January–February), pp. 59–67.

SORKIN, A. L. (1975) *Health Economics*. Lexington, Massachusetts: Lexington Books, D. C. Heath & Co.

WILSON, R. W. and WHITE, E. L. (1977) 'Changes in Morbidity, Disability and Utilisation Differentials between the Poor and the Nonpoor: Data from the Health Interview Survey, 1964 and 1973', *Medical Care*, Vol. 15, No. 8 (August), pp. 636–46.

12 Economic Aspects of a Developing Health Care System

> . . . some [political leaderships] lack the will to challenge the enormous inequalities of their societies even in the cause of better health for the majority . . . . The contribution to the health of Western nations of their costly and prestigious hospitals has been small compared to the introduction and use of clean water, the safe disposal of excreta, higher standards of personal hygiene and improved nutrition.
>
> *B. Abel-Smith* (1976, pp. 195–6)

12.1 Introduction

This book has so far analysed a wide range of arguments that suggest that the allocation of health care resources in developed countries could be improved. The search for such improvements in a developing country is made crucially important by the scarcity of health care resources relative to the massive scale of health problems that they face. Developing countries suffer infant mortality rates ten to twenty times greater than those in developed countries, and endemic infectious diseases[1] that cripple the individual and the economy. Yet their health service budgets are one-hundredth the *per capita* size of those in developed countries. Medical manpower and hospital facilities are constrained by these small budgets to the order of one-fifteenth of European levels of provision (World Health Organisation, 1971), and even these slender resources are distributed with enormous inequity.

Large urban hospitals, designed to provide 'Western' acute care for colonial rulers, have been preserved to service the equally privileged élites in developing countries. Where such hospitals require a fee for service, their location and mix of services necessarily reflects the pattern of effective demand and income distribution. Hospital location concentrates expenditure in centres inaccessible to the rural population, who typically face a long and physically taxing journey to the cities when relatively healthy, an impossible journey when ill. Yet urban hospitals continue to absorb resources disproportionately (see Tables 12.1 and 12.2) while providing treatment largely for the local community only (e.g., 80 per cent

Table 12.1 Analysis of Government Health Expenditures in Selected Countries

Country	Year	Total public expenditures ($ million)	Percentage for public health or prevention	Percentage for curative care	Percentage for training and research
Sri Lanka	1957–58	34.3	23.3	74.4	2.3
Tanzania	1970–71	19.5	4.9	80.3	4.4
India	1965–66	236.0	37.0	55.5	7.5
Laos[a]	1971–72	2.3	14.3[b]	19.9[c]	44.8
Kenya	1971	27.8	5.2	83.8	11.0
Thailand[a]	1971–72	83.6	28.1[d]	46.6[c]	19.1
Paraguay[a]	1972	10.0	10.5[e]	8.46[c]	—
Tunisia[a]	1971	15.8	—	86.3[c]	—
El Salvador[a]	1971	30.4	3.3[f]	52.9[c]	1.1
Turkey[a]	1972	303.7	16.3[g]	—	13.5
Colombia	1970	203.0	18.7	79.3	2.0
Mongolia[a]	1972	—	—	—	7.2
Chile	1959	63.8	18.3	77.0	4.0
Panama	1967	28.4	30.0	70	
Venezuela	1962	—	18.0	76.5	5.5
Israel[d]	1959–60	82.7	4.9	80.3	4.4

[a] Classification of residual categories of expenditure is unknown
[b] Expenditure for 'environmental health services'
[c] Expenditure for government hospitals only
[d] Expenditure for 'control of communicable diseases, laboratory services, environmental health services and occupational health services'
[e] Expenditure for 'campaign against communicable diseases, maternal and child health and vaccinations and laboratory services'
[f] Expenditure for 'immunisation and vaccination activities, laboratory services and environmental health services'
[g] Expenditure for 'mass campaigns against communicable diseases, immunisation and vaccination activities, laboratory services and environmental health services'

Source: World Bank (1975, Annex 4)

Table 12.2 Percentage Distribution of Health Expenditures in Selected Countries, 1961

Country	Personal medical services In-patient (%)	Personal medical services Out-patient (%)	Public health services (%)	Teaching and research (%)
Kenya	89		8	3
Sri Lanka	50	44	5	2
Tanzania	45	50	4	1
Yugoslavia	43	50	4	3
Czechoslovakia	48	44	2	6
United Kingdom	52	44	2	2
France	41	56	2	2
Sweden	53	42	1	4
United States	38	57	1	5

Source: World Bank (1975, Annex 5)

of patients at a new hospital in Uganda were drawn from the 20 per cent of the population living in the neighbouring area: ITDG, 1971). Such figures would be equitable only if there were many such hospitals, each serving a small area. Where there are very few, hospitals concentrate the use of resources and leave the mass of the population with virtually no health care facilities.

The scale of the health budget in developing countries and the extent to which it is pre-empted by hospitals raises the fundamental question of the choice of technique to be used to combat health problems. The balance between curative and preventative services currently favours the former in many developing countries, but there is a growing awareness that such emphasis is inappropriate. Indeed, many observers of countries such as China, which have coupled preventive measures with paramedic barefoot doctor schemes, have posed similar questions about the balance of resource use in developed countries.

In the discussion that follows, we concentrate on three aspects of health and health services in developing countries. These are (a) the links between health and development, (b) the evaluation of alternative uses of health service resources and their implications for policy, and (c) the manpower problems of developing health systems. Having reviewed these dimensions of the problem, we then consider their implications for the future development of health services in developing countries.

12.2 Health and development

The state of health of the population of a developing country and its rate of economic development are related in two ways. While development provides the possibility for improved health by permitting greater expenditure on health, there are equally strong causal links from health to development. As noted in Chapter 2, improved health increases the effective labour force by cutting debility, disability and mortality. Low levels of nutrition reduce productivity by damaging physical and mental health from conception onwards. The poor remuneration paid in return for the reduced work effort in its turn prevents improved nutrition and effectively completes an entrapping chain of deprivation. The available evidence suggests that, if this chain could be broken, the potential economic gains would be considerable. Thus, Basta and Churchill (1974) found a ratio of benefits to costs of 260 : 1 for a programme of diet supplementation with iron for malnourished workers, (though whether similar scales of benefit would result from a given programme depends on existing nutrition levels and constituents e.g. see Scrimshaw *et al.* (1968)).

Attempts have also been made to evaluate the contribution of improved health to productivity by regression analysis of the growth of output. Malenbaum (1970) found in a study of twenty-two countries that health variables accounted for over three-quarters of the 62 per cent explained variance in agricultural output (though his model and data have been criticised by Weisbrod *et al.*, 1973). Similarly Griffith *et al.* (1971), again using regression analysis, found that output per worker was more than twice as responsive to health expenditure per worker as to the share of GNP invested in capital. But aside from reservations about the quality of data used in such studies, the further difficulty is that regression analysis does not separate out the two directions of causality, from health expenditure to income and from income to health expenditure.[2]

The increased output of a healthy worker is by no means the sole economic benefit. The very high mortality rates for children in developing countries mean that food supplies are partly used to support individuals who never reach the work force. Putting aside the toll of human misery that such mortality brings, it has been estimated by Berg (1973) that 20 per cent of Indian national income prior to independence was absorbed in feeding children who subsequently died without reaching the labour force. Reduced mortality for the young would thus reduce the economic loss and increase the future work force.

The effects of improved health on development are complicated, however, by the changes in population that result. The benefits of development may be eroded by subsequent population increases, particularly if opportunities for using the additional work force to increase output are limited. The 'Iron Law of Wages', propounded in the nineteenth century in Europe, suggested that wage rates above subsistence level would lead to growth in family size, owing in part to the greater infant survival rates. This depresses *per capita* consumption back to subsistence level, the only long-run equilibrium possible. Clearly, there is a sense in which this law is definitionally true. In the period immediately following the reduction in infant mortality the larger number of surviving children consume without contributing, except perhaps very marginally, to production. But the very long-run accuracy of its prediction is more difficult to assess. The growth of the work force (and dependants) may exceed the growth of total output if marginal productivity is low owing to constraints on the resources and capital available for production. However, if increased survival affects fertility rates, the rate of growth of population will slow. This will reduce the proportion of dependants, mainly children, in the population and so will offset, at least partially, the decline in *per capita* consumption.

It is difficult to generalise from Western experience of rising living standards to determine the necessary conditions for similar improvements in developing countries (though the late arrival of medicine in the West suggests that its contribution was small). Cultural values and ignorance may militate against reductions in family size and, in the absence of widespread education and contraceptive advice, are likely to prove the more dominant influences. Furthermore, attempts to evaluate the long-run consequences of health improvements on development are fraught with difficulties.

Detailed studies of the effects of population growth on *per capita* income and consumption highlight the adverse consequences of population growth for investment in particular. Meade (1967) and Barlow (1967, 1968) have examined the effects of relatively rapid population growth for confined areas, the islands of Mauritius and Sri Lanka. Meade demonstrated the links between consumption and population growth with a simple fixed-coefficient model of production. Assume that output per worker will remain constant as the labour force expands only if the capital-to-labour ratio remains constant. Thus, if the population (and work force) grows at a rate (n) per year, required investment in new capital ($\bar{I}$) must equal a proportion (n) of the total capital stock (K). Meade suggested that the capital stock of a developing country would be approximately four times its annual GNP (Y). Formally, if

$$K = 4 \tag{12.1}$$

then

$$\bar{I} = nK = 4nY. \tag{12.2}$$

That is, for every percentage point rise in the population growth rate, an increase of four percentage points in the share of GNP invested in new capital is required to maintain output per head. Therefore consumption per head is lower in an economy with a fast growing population even when output per head is maintained. Since it is likely that the propensity to consume will be close to one for the poor, any cut in aggregate consumption is likely to require a reduction in their income either directly or through the lowering of wages to increase the return on investment and the saving of the rich.

Barlow has attempted a detailed macro-evaluation of the effect of health improvement on the long-run economic development of a developing country. Sri Lanka (formerly Ceylon) experienced a substantial decline in mortality in the immediate postwar period. Much of this has been attributed to a programme to eradicate malaria on the island, though whether this was the major cause has been the subject of extensive debate (see e.g. Frederiksen, 1960, 1961; Gray, 1974). Barlow focused on income *per capita* and attempted to develop an econometric model that would simulate the growth path of income *per capita* in the absence of the decline in mortality. In so far as the decline in mortality was due to the elimination of malaria, a number of economic aspects of the impact of the disease are relevant. Malaria is a disease against which the individual can protect himself by a variety of precautions such as location of housing, sleeping under netting and by prophylactic medication. Furthermore, treatment of malaria with drugs is likely to reduce the consequences of any infection that occurs. However, the costs of these precautions and the education necessary to encourage them mean that higher-income groups take more steps to counter the disease, and its incidence becomes income-related. Barlow argued that, since the eradication of malaria impinged on low-income groups, the economic benefits were less to the extent that such groups had low productivity (even when healthy). However, the links between productivity and income distribution may be affected by the ownership of land, concentration of which could lead to low incomes for landless peasants and an income below their marginal product (economic exploitation).

Central to Barlow's analysis was a Cobb – Douglas production function linking labour of different kinds with capital and output. Labour was separated into skilled and unskilled and each was quality-weighted to allow for differential productivity. Similarly, a quality weight was placed on capital inputs to reflect the mixture of productive and social capital. As the population of any country grows, more investment is required for housing, schools, etc. and so less is put into investment yielding direct production benefits. Thus, the quality index was reduced as population increased. Formally,

$$Q = q_1 L_1^{\alpha} q_2 L_2^{\beta} q_3 K^{\gamma} \qquad (12.3)$$

where q_1, q_2, q_3 are quality weights on skilled and unskilled labour and capital; Q is total output; L_1, L_2 are skilled and unskilled labour inputs; K is capital input and α, β, γ are exponents of the production function. The reader familiar with such production functions will be aware that, when the sum of the exponents equals one, the exponents indicate the share of total output going to each input (which receives its marginal product as a wage or price).[3]

By using data on existing income shares to estimate α, β, γ, and by taking medical opinions on the labour quality weight with and without malaria, Barlow was able to simulate output in the absence of the malaria eradication. The other equations in the model permit the estimation of various key economic variables.

The most notable of the estimated results concerns consumption and saving *per capita*. Barlow's simulations suggested that up to 1955 consumption *per capita* was higher owing to the eradication of malaria. But the adverse effects of more rapid population growth had already taken their toll on saving, and hence investment, by this time; e.g., by 1953 government saving was substantially lower than it would have been without rapid population growth.

Such predictions as these are obviously sensitive to the particular assumptions of the model. For example, Borts (1967) has criticised Barlow's assumption of fixed exports. Growth in export revenue would permit greater overseas borrowing and would offset the decline in investment, at least partially, and so reduce the impact of population growth. But regardless of the particular assumptions made, Barlow's work demonstrated that the results of improved health are not unambiguous.

One final, and fundamental, effect of population growth concerns the distribution of income. Improved health and a growing work force may depress wages in spite of higher productivity. Furthermore, low wages and a high return on capital may be necessary to encourage investment from both internal and external sources. Thus, improved health may not improve living standards for the mass of the population even when GNP *per capita* is rising (e.g., recent evidence quoted by Bavandi (1975) suggests that the share of GNP going to the poorest sections of the population is declining in most developing countries).

12.3 Preventive versus curative approaches

A major difficulty confronting any attempt to allocate health service resources efficiently in a developing country is the absence of data on the benefits of particular forms of treatment or prevention.

Barlow (1976) has attempted to remedy this by estimating the costs of saving lives under alternative health care strategies in order to provide a guide for health planning policy in Morocco. A comparison was made of vaccination and hospital treatment as alternative methods of dealing with tuberculosis, smallpox, diphtheria and other infectious diseases.

Any attempt to identify the outcomes of these approaches faces a severe research problem in determining the life-saving effects of hospitals and injections. It can be tackled in at least two ways. The first is to examine the correlation between mortality from a given disease and hospital admission. Clearly, if the majority of patients hospitalised with a particular disease survive while sufferers outside hospital do not it is tempting to infer that the hospital is the cause of any reduction in mortality. However, in a developing country there is likely to be a number of differences between the population treated in hospital and that outside. Income is likely to be an important factor determining whether an individual receives hospital care that is not provided free of user charges. Since income will also correlate with nutrition, education and access to hospitals, it is likely that survival rates will also be correlated with income, thus biasing upwards the hospital survival statistics. The alternative technique, which avoids this bias and was preferred for that reason by Barlow, involves a case-by-case assessment to identify the effect of hospital care on the probability of death within one year. Clearly, the findings of such investigations are affected by the particular experts assessing these probabilities, but this bias is unavoidable and acceptable given the limitations of the other method. Similar estimates were constructed by Barlow indicating the lives saved per injection.

The estimated costs of hospital care and vaccination were combined with the probabilistic estimates of lives saved to yield the cost per life saved by each technique. Barlow's results gave a cost per life saved by vaccination of 120 dirhams for tuberculosis, 190 dirhams for diphtheria, tetanus and whooping cough (a combined injection) and 5500 dirhams for polio. Even the very much higher figure for polio vaccination compares favourably with the cost of hospital care, estimated at between 11,000 and 15,000 dirhams per life saved. Thus, although subject to reservations about the degree of accuracy of its findings, Barlow's research clearly indicates the relative merits of prevention. In view of the reduced suffering associated with preventive measures, the advantages of vaccination seem overwhelming.

However, the strength of the case for vaccination is only a part of the argument for concentration on preventive measures to improve population health. Medicine, even in the form of vaccinations, was not the major cause of reductions in death rates in Western Europe in the period 1800–1950. Of itself, this does not imply that medicine cannot provide solutions for developing countries. Its success in eliminating infectious diseases already in decline in Europe suggests that it can destroy infecting organisms almost at a stroke. For example, a global campaign aimed at eliminating smallpox has led to its virtual disappearance. Only small areas, and very small numbers of people, now face the threat of this once widely spread disease. But to focus on the success of any single medical programme aimed at rendering the world's population free from a given organism ignores the major weaknesses of such programmes. First, the vaccination is specific to only one disease in an environment where individuals face a multitude of different threats to health. Second, organisms can develop immunity to vaccination and other specific preventive measures. The main advantage of direct public health measures is that, by disrupting the mechanism of disease communication, they eradicate a range of disorders simultaneously. Furthermore, there are a number of diseases that contribute considerably to mortality but do not respond to treatment or vaccination. Pneumonia and gastroenteric diseases have been highlighted by Bryant (1969), for example, as typical of disorders that are major causes of mortality among the young and for which no effective prophylaxis exists.

A further advantage of preventive measures that aim at physical alteration of the environment or education to modify individual behaviour is that they may be less costly than even vaccination programmes. Their cost advantage falls into two categories, direct cost and foreign exchange costs. Environment modification is frequently labour-intensive, and so by drawing on the local population it can avoid making claims on the limited health budget. Although its use of labour may not be entirely costless, co-ordination of the work with periods of relative inactivity in the agricultural cycle can reduce such costs by minimising the disruption of other work effort. Modification of individual behaviour, e.g. sanitatary measures, may also involve little cost beyond initial education programmes, though the success of such behaviour-modifying activities will depend closely on factors such as the general level of education and frequency of reinforcement.

Foreign exchange costs may be of central importance where drugs and vaccines have to be imported in finished or raw material form. Gish (1975) has suggested that the cost of pharmaceutical products accounts for around 25 per cent of the health budget of African countries. While much of this would be absorbed by the hospital sector, it is noteworthy that individual vaccines, e.g. against measles, may be too costly for developing countries to use on a mass scale in spite of the high levels of mortality among measles sufferers in developing countries (Office of Health Economics, 1972). The use of foreign exchange for health programmes will be heavily constrained by the competing claims for capital equipment necessary to provide the infrastructure for economic growth. Thus its shadow price may raise the costs of vaccination and reduce the coverage of vaccination programmes even when at face value they are highly cost-effective.

Paradoxically, as Abel-Smith (1976) has pointed out, the developed countries would secure considerable direct gain from the elimination of some infectious diseases in developing countries. It is common in developed countries for costly vaccinations to be given on a regular basis to large sections of the population, especially travellers. Although total expenditures on such vaccinations are not known for all countries, they have been estimated to be as high as $150 million for smallpox alone in the USA in 1968. If expenditures on this scale in the developed world could be avoided by successful eradication programmes, they would ironically outweigh the direct tangible benefits in the form of averted expenditures on smallpox secured by developing nations. Despite such potential gains that developed countries ought on a benefit principle to be willing to finance, it is generally the case that developing countries are constrained to use the resources that they possess themselves. The main resource is labour, much of which is located in rural areas.

The Republic of China provides perhaps the best example of mobilisation of the rural population *en masse* and emphasis on rural programmes to achieve health improvements. As early as 1952 China had instituted 'Patriotic Health Campaigns' using mass participation to eradicate rats, flies, mosquitoes and bedbugs, and to improve the quality of water supplies. The wide popular involvement not only contributed to the success of these and subsequent schemes, but also provided scope for health education to increase public awareness of the mechanisms of disease transmission. Health was also integrated into the broader economic plans for agriculture which became the focus for aspirations of economic growth in the late 1950s. The large rural work force was viewed as the major resource on which agricultural development was to be based. This reinforced the emphasis on rural health services and discouraged over-concentration on urban-based technological medicine. Urban hospital doctors now spend periods of time working in rural areas, not only to provide treatment but also to train paramedics at various levels and to be reminded forcefully of the importance of the rural economy and its health needs. This is not to suggest that China has ignored the development of a hospital system. A network of hospitals from small one- or two-man clinics to urban specialist hospitals exists throughout the country. But primary emphasis is placed on the 'barefoot doctor' who provides low-technology medicine for everyday ailments and health education focused on prevention.

The reduced emphasis on technological medicine has been assisted by the survival in China of traditional medicine alongside Western 'scientific' medicine. Acupuncture is widely used as an anaesthetic, for example, in major operations of a highly sophisticated kind. Herbal remedies may be preferred by the rural population instead of modern drugs, thus reducing the cost of health care. By contrast, the monopoly power of medical practitioners in developed countries leads them constantly to seek sanctions against any 'non-scientific' methods that represent competition to this monopoly. Thus, homeopathy for example has virtually disappeared from health services in Britain. The absence of such a powerful monopoly in China has also brought greater flexibility into health care programmes, e.g. teachers have been trained to give injections against diseases such as tuberculosis in order to reduce the manpower required for mass coverage vaccination schemes.

In spite of its mass health campaigns, there are general reservations about the success of health programmes in China. Reliable evidence on the incidence of particular diseases is not readily available and so it is difficult to evaluate the achievements of China's preventive and educational measures. Huang (1973) in reviewing the ten major diseases of modern China has suggested that, in spite of widespread popular involvement in education and public health, many of these disorders are not yet under control. Preventive measures against, e.g., schistosomiasis have been in operation for more than twenty years but have done little to reduce the areas of the country where the disease is endemic (and irrigation projects, which can spread the disease, have increased its prevalence in some places). Similarly, attempts to control the eye disease trachoma by encouraging public awareness of its transmission mechanisms (shared towels and washing water), together with mobile units and stations for detection and treatment, have apparently achieved only limited success.

It seems legitimate, therefore, to conclude that the development of improved health in developing countries is by no means a short and simple process. Preventive and public health measures may be successful where the level of public awareness is high. Vaccination and therapy may also be effective where they have been developed. But all four measures are only of limited effect in the short run when attempting to counter many endemic diseases that affect a rural population that in most developing countries is undernourished. However, the comparative costs of these different approaches to the health budget is likely to continue to make public and preventive health measures the suitable weapons of health policy in developing countries.

Before leaving this section, it is worth noting that it is sometimes possible to combine curative and preventive medicine by, for example, using mobile clinics whose staff, in the process of treating the sick, can also provide vaccinations and advice on health education to those within needle and ear shot. Although this may be the logical approach on economic grounds, political constraints may well bind the selection of preventive as opposed to curative measures. As Abel-Smith (1976) has pointed out, political pressure may create a bias towards curative medicine because the results are clearly seen to follow (with a short time lag) the action taken. Hence preventive health policies, which may not be readily comprehended but have high long-term 'pay-offs', may be sacrificed on the altar of political expediency for smaller short-run gains.

Finally, in any comparison of alternative methods of securing widespread health improvements from limited resources, the difficulty of identifying causal relationships cannot be overlooked. Returning to the decline in mortality in Sri Lanka, the available data challenge the links between eradication of malaria and declining mortality.

12.4 Manpower and developing health care systems

The discussion throughout this chapter has emphasised the relative advantages of concentration on public health and preventive measures in developing countries. This in turn implies that medical education in Western medicine to Western standards (apart from public health measures) is largely inappropriate. However, there are a number of features of the supply of medical manpower in developing countries that may frustrate the successful introduction of large numbers of less highly trained medical aides.

Some developing countries currently train large numbers of medical practitioners themselves in university medical schools. However, as a result of the setting of medical and educational standards in the era of colonial rule, these doctors are trained in large part to practise highly sophisticated Western medicine rather than more elementary preventive medicine, and consequently they absorb large amounts of any training budgets. On qualifying, they naturally seek to practise what they have learnt in urban hospitals and so their services are unlikely to affect the major health problems of the rural population. Furthermore, aside from the nature of their work, there are also economic incentives favouring urban hospital practice. Pay and conditions are likely to be much better in the services of a privileged urban élite – those who can afford both Western diseases and the subsequent health care required – who offer scope for private practice in addition to regular employment.

Economic incentives may also lead medical manpower to quit the developing countries completely for the higher salaries and living standards of developed countries. The UK has in the recent past come to depend heavily on immigrant doctors from Commonwealth countries such as India and Pakistan. By the late 1960s 15,200 foreign-born doctors, amounting to 22 per cent of the total supply, were practising in Britain, and over half of these had trained in the Commonwealth countries of Asia (Gish, 1971). Many are in the UK ostensibly for further training through experience as junior hospital doctors, but this is questionable in that the value of such training in a development context is very limited. Rather, they now fill the gaps in Britain's medical manpower owing to migration, undersupply or career choice by domestic doctors.

Although largely trained before arrival in the UK, Asian doctors have been to a considerable extent treated much as migrant workers in most developed economies. They are channelled into the less interesting or rewarding specialties which British doctors are less inclined to choose. At the time of Gish's research 88 per cent of hospital posts at the grade of registrar in geriatric medicine were held by immigrants compared with 30 per cent in the more scientific discipline of radiology. This not only affects the type of 'training' that they receive from their work experience, but also restricts their access to income from private practice. However, even these drawbacks to immigration have failed to reverse the trend from Asia to Europe. And when immigrants do return they are more likely to practise privately or in urban hospitals since their experience in Britain will have provided little of use in a rural setting (Gish, 1975) (e.g., geriatric medicine is of little use when infant mortality is the major health problem).

Clearly, the flow of medical manpower represents substantial transfers of resources from poor training countries to rich receiving countries (estimated at £150 million for doctors currently in the UK: Office of Health Economics, 1972). The offsetting loss of UK doctors to Europe and North America can be no consolation to developing countries. Why then do developing countries continue to provide training that is not only inappropriate for their own needs but that provides the trained medical manpower with an entrée to developed countries? Pressure to reduce the flow has if anything been stronger from within the UK, with the recent introduction of examinations for new immigrant doctors. The answer probably lies in a complex interaction of factors such as status and clinical standards in the medical schools of developing countries. The medical profession of such countries is unlikely to permit the undermining of its position both internally and externally by a lowering of standards, which might reflect adversely on those already trained. For example, the Pakistan medical profession abandoned the grade of licentiate following the rejection of such a qualification for entry into UK medical practice by the General Medical Council (Office of Health Economics, 1972). Similarly, rising academic standards have further shifted the pattern of medical training away from the requirements of the rural sector. Gish (1971) has noted the effects of academic 'overkill' which lead trained medical auxiliaries to pursue further training rather than return to rural health care services. Thus we can observe the effects of economic incentives and intellectual aspirations throughout the hierarchy of world medicine. The pinnacle of medical practice is represented by the urban specialist hospital. Western technological medicine, in which considerably less rigorous budget constraints permit the practice of medicine with little regard to cost, is preferred to rural practice with few resources and little chance of financial success. Only where the pressures for movement towards the Western medical mode are removed can effective rural health manpower be provided on a sufficient scale.

The Republic of China has again been most successful in this respect, establishing a widespread network of so-called 'barefoot doctors' or, more accurately, rural health auxiliaries. The scale of this network, with a village of 200 people having perhaps two or three such aides, permits the successful combination of medical and agricultural work. (A typical general practitioner in the UK provides primary care for 2000–3000 people.) Only a few months of training is required to teach the barefoot doctor the elementary treatment of routine cases and the recognition of cases requiring referral. This may appear remarkably short in comparison with the five years of medical training in the UK, for example, but it is merely a facet of the division of labour utilised by the Chinese but frustrated by the medical profession in most developed and many developing countries. In a developed country, primary contact with a five-year trained medical practitioner is largely unnecessary since the bulk of diseases are relatively trivial and self-limiting. As long as the first contact in the medical chain is given clear guidelines on what he treats and what he refers to a more highly trained medical practitioner, only brief training is required. In other words, it is not necessary for the medical auxiliary to have detailed knowledge of every possible disease. All that is required is a set of fail-safe criteria which ensure that he refers any extraordinary cases. Of course, mis-diagnosis may occur, but the costs of avoiding it are likely to be prohibitive. Furthermore, since in many developing countries there are few resources to treat the complex disorders, the main advantage of a highly educated primary care practitioner is effectively negated.

Again, it is not possible to evaluate the advantages and disadvantages of medical manpower schemes that aim for quantity rather than sophistication. But the cost differences between the various levels of medical hierarchy from barefoot doctor to teaching hospital professor are such that differences in their success in the field would need to be enormous if highly trained doctors were to emerge as the major type of manpower for rural health. Furthermore, since for many of the diseases facing the mass of the population in developing countries effective treatments are relatively simple, the pattern of disease itself makes sophistication largely unnecessary.

12.5 Health care policy – an alternative approach

In the absence of any clear evidence of the 'best buy' in health services for developing countries and the presence of what appear to be gross misallocation of resources between rich and poor, city and country, the economist's role is perhaps less technical in a development context. The multi-dimensional nature of the pattern of sickness in developing countries makes attempts to isolate the costs and benefits of a single health measure of limited usefulness. Conversely, the current distribution of income is so clearly inappropriate in many developing countries that its further analysis seems of little relevance. However, the economist can still make a contribution to the planning of health services less by calculating the optimal amount of each service required than by laying bare the policy options available to the health planner. A fixed budget and existing manpower can be used to implement a range of alternative projects from public health to hospital building. Only by setting out the options and monitoring the progress to particular objectives can the health planner learn from past events and improve future performance.

It is of course the policy-maker's task to determine the targets of the health plan.[4] The economist's role is then to identify as far as possible (and this may not be all that far) the cost-effective means to achieving the desired goals. At its most basic this may mean simply identifying the opportunity cost of individual activities since the absence of data is a major hurdle in the path to the best health plan. More fundamentally however, the economist should be combining with other experts to identify the significant features that have led to successful health programmes in the past. The importance of community participation leads to the inclusion of sociologists and educationists in any health planning teams together with doctors and epidemiologists. Ultimately it will be their success in creating programmes that are inexpensive, culturally acceptable and effective that will determine actual health improvements within the potential created by changes in the amount and the distribution of food and income (see Gish, 1975, and WHO, 1977).

12.6 Summary

In this chapter we have explored three aspects of resource allocation in a developing health care system. Concerning the first, it was argued that the relationship between health and development, as with most economic mechanisms, is a complex one. The major difficulty is that improved health, by increasing the growth rate of the population, in the short run puts greater pressure on scarce food supplies, and even in the long run may not raise living standards owing to diminishing returns to labour.

The use of scarce health service resources and meagre budgets is obviously of crucial importance, and it was argued that such resources should be focused in particular on preventive care and public health measures both to achieve a more effective outcome and to avoid the pitfalls of the technological medicine 'rat race'.

Finally, it was argued that manpower programmes should also concentrate on the less sophisticated aspects of medicine in order to provide the widest possible coverage of primary care.

Of course it would be unrealistic to regard these arguments as forming a complete panacea for health problems in developing countries. Indeed, the links between nutrition and health in such countries make it essential that any health policy be part of a broadly based programme of action. But none the less, it is our view that the best buy in health services for developing countries lies not in the high-technology industrial model, the problems of which have been amply demonstrated throughout this book, but in a low-technology mass-based and predominantly preventive health care system.

NOTES

1. For a description of the main sources of ill health in developing countries see Chapter 1, n.4.
2. The limited evidence presented in Section 1.5 above is consistent with the causality running from income to health expenditure. Government health expenditures *per capita* were found to have an income elasticity greater than unity.
3. Formally, the marginal product of e.g. skilled labour is:

$$\frac{\partial Q}{\partial L_1} = \alpha q_1 L_1^{\alpha-1} q_2 L_2^{\beta} q_3 K^{\gamma}$$

$$= \frac{\alpha Q}{L_1}.$$

$$= \alpha Q.$$

$$\therefore\ Y_1 = \frac{\partial Q}{\partial L_1} \cdot L_1$$

Therefore, skilled labour receives a share of total output equal to α:

$$\frac{Y_1}{Q} = \alpha.$$

4. It is to be remembered however that developing countries often lack the necessary expertise. For example, Ugalde (1978) points out that in Iran 'National health planners were never taken very seriously by top decision makers because of the former's lack of expertise in health planning: e.g. cost-benefit and cost-efficiency analysis, or budgeting programs by cost, was beyond their capabilities' (p. 2).

REFERENCES

ABEL-SMITH, B. (1976) *Value for Money in Health Services.* London: Heinemann.

BARLOW, R. (1967) 'The Economic Effect of Malaria Eradication', *American Economic Review* (Papers and Proceedings), Vol. 57, No. 2 (May), pp. 130–48.

BARLOW, R. (1968) *The Economic Effects of Malaria Eradication* (Research Series No. 15). Ann Arbor, Michigan: Bureau of Public Health Economics.

BARLOW, R. (1976) 'Application of a Health Planning Model in Morocco, *International Journal of Health Services,* Vol. 6, No. 1 (February), pp. 103–22.

BASTA, S. S. and CHURCHILL, A. (1974) 'Iron Deficiency Anaemia and the Productivity of Adult Males in Indonesia', *Staff Working Paper No. 173, Research Division* (Transport and Urban Projects Department). Washington DC: International Bank for Reconstruction and Development.

BAVANDI, M. (1975) 'Industrial Growth and Nutrition', *Health and Industrial Growth* (CIBA Foundation Symposium 32). Amsterdam: North Holland, Elsevier, Excerpta Medica.

BERG, A. (1973) *The Nutrition Factor: Its Role in National Development.* Washington DC: Brookings Institution.

BORTS, G. H. (1967) 'The Economic Effect of Malaria Eradication: Discussion', *American Economic Review* (Papers and Proceedings), Vol. 57, No. 2 (May), p. 149.

BRYANT, J. (1969) *Health and the Developing World.* Ithaca, New York: Cornell University Press.

FREDERIKSEN, H. (1960) 'Malaria Control and Population Pressure in Ceylon', *Public Health Reports*, Vol. 75, No. 10 (October), pp. 865–8.

FREDERIKSEN, H. (1961) 'Determinants and Consequences of Mortality Trends in Ceylon', *Public Health Reports*, Vol. 76, No. 8 (August), pp. 659–63.

GISH, O. (1971) *Doctor Migration and World Health* (Occasional Papers on Social Administration, No. 43). London: Bell.

GISH, O. (1975) *Planning the Health Sector: The Tanzanian Experience.* London: Croom Helm.

GRAY, R. H. (1974) 'Decline in Mortality in Ceylon and the Demographic Effects of Malaria Control,' *Population Studies*, Vol. 28, No. 2 (July), pp. 205–30.

GRIFFITH, D. H. S., RAMANA, D. V. and MASHAAL, A. (1971) 'Contribution of Health to Development,' *International Journal of Health Services* Vol. 1, No. 3 (August), pp. 253–70.

HUANG, K.-Y. (1973) 'Infectious and Parasitic Diseases', pp. 263–88 in Quinn, J. R. (ed.) *Medicine and Public Health in the People's Republic of China.* Bethesda: John E. Fogarty International Centre for Advanced Study in the Health Sciences.

INTERNATIONAL TECHNOLOGY DEVELOPMENT GROUP (1971) *Health Manpower and the Health Auxiliary.* London: I.T.D.G.

MALENBAUM, W. (1970) 'Health and Productivity in Poor Areas', pp. 31–54 in Klarman, H. (ed.) *Empirical Studies in Health Economics.* Baltimore: Johns Hopkins.

MEADE, J. E. (1967) 'Population Explosion, the Standard of Living and Social Conflict', *Economic Journal*, Vol. 77, No. 306 (June), pp. 233–55.

OFFICE OF HEALTH ECONOMICS (1972) *Medical Care in Developing Countries* (Studies on Current Health Problems, No. 44). London: OHE.

SCRIMSHAW, N. S., *et al.* (1968) 'Nutrition and Infection Field Study in Guatemalan Villages, 1959–64', *Archives of Environmental Health*, Vol. 18, (January), pp. 51–62.

UGALDE, A. (1978) 'Health Decision Making in Developing Nations: A Comparative Analysis of Columbia and Iran', *Social Science and Medicine*, Vol. 12, No. 1A (January), pp. 1–7.

WEISBROD, B. *et al.* (1973) *Disease and Economic Development: The Impact of Parasitic Diseases in St Lucia.* Madison, Wisconsin: University of Wisconsin Press.

WORLD BANK (1975) *Health* (Sector Policy Paper), March. Washington DC: World Bank.

WORLD HEALTH ORGANISATION (1971) *Fourth Report on World Health Situation 1965–68.* Geneva: WHO.

Some Suggested Essay Questions

1. 'Health care is a "necessity" and as such should be allocated resources irrespective of any considerations of cost and benefit.' Discuss.

2. 'It seems we have to view health care as a consumption good in both developed and developing countries.' Give reasons for agreeing or disagreeing with this statement and indicate how you might analyse health care as a consumption good.

3. 'The characteristics that make health care "different" do not imply that one method of provision is superior to another.' Discuss.

4. Assess the importance of 'giving' and 'sharing' as motives for setting up the British NHS.

5. In Grossman's model of the demand for health individuals 'choose' their length of life. What is meant by this? Do you see any connection between the Grossman approach to the demand for health care and one based on the notion of 'need'?

6. Indicate some of the problems in estimating demand elasticities for health care. What is the policy relevance of the results reported to date?

7. 'Economic models of hospitals are elegant but yield few important implications for public policy.' Discuss.

8. 'Empirical evidence on the shape of hospital cost functions is so varied as to be useless.' Discuss.

9. 'The difficulties of applying cost – benefit and cost-effectiveness analysis in the field of health care are so great that analyses carried out to date provide no important insights regarding the choice of alternatives.' Do you agree?

10. Imagine you are a professional economist called as an expert witness in a court case and the judge asks you how the problem of valuing human life is tackled by economists. What is your reply; what is the approach with which the judge would be familiar; and which, if any, is right?

11. 'The problems with the American medical care system stem from "too much market", whereas the problems of the British National Health Service stem from "too much state".' What are the problems? Do you agree with the diagnoses?

12. Do the health care problems of developing countries differ from those in developed countries? If so, why so; how so?

Suggested Further Reading

General. The Economics of Health

Other texts on the economics of health are relatively few. Two books that include a wide range of material are Berki (1972) and Culyer (1976). The former is more sophisticated in terms of economics and is American, while the latter relates to the National Health Service and is by design aimed at the social science generalist rather than the economics specialist. An article-length treatment of the economics of health that includes an extensive bibliography with 'key' items emphasised is provided by Williams (1977). A useful book of readings, now beginning to 'date' slightly but nevertheless including many 'classics', is Cooper and Culyer (1973). Other fairly recent works exclusively devoted to health economics are Fuchs (1972), (1974), Hauser (1972) and Perlman (1974). Daedalus (1977) is devoted to papers on all aspects of the American health care system. Culyer, Wiseman and Walker (1977) is an annotated bibliography of health economics English language sources up to 1974. A very recent collection of papers on the economics of health services largely in the UK is Culyer and Wright (1978). Finally, Weeks and Berman (1977) is a valuable collection of thirty major health economics papers published in the eleven years since 1966 in the Blue Cross Association's journal *Inquiry*.

BERKI, S. E. (1972) *Hospital Economics.* Lexington, Massachusetts: Lexington Books, D. C. Heath & Co.

COOPER, M. H. and CULYER, A. J. (1973) *Health Economics.* Harmondsworth: Penguin.

CULYER, A. J. (1976) *Need and the National Health Service: Economics and Social Choice.* London: Martin Robertson.

CULYER, A. J., WISEMAN, J. and WALKER, A. (1977) *An Annotated Bibliography of Health Economics English Language Sources.* London: Martin Robertson.

CULYER, A. J. and WRIGHT, K. G. (1978) *Economic Aspects of Health Services.* London: Martin Robertson.

DAEDALUS (1977) *Doing Better and Feeling Worse: Health in the United States* (Proceedings of American Academy of Arts and Sciences), Vol. 106, No. 1 (Winter).

FUCHS, V. R. (ed.) (1972) *Essays in the Economics of Health and Medical Care*. New York and London: Columbia University Press for National Bureau of Economic Research.

FUCHS, V. R. (1974) *Who Shall Live? Health, Economics and Social Choice*. New York: Basic Books.

HAUSER, M. M. (ed.), (1972) *The Economics of Medical Care*. London: George Allen & Unwin.

PERLMAN, M. (ed.) (1974) *The Economics of Health and Medical Care*. London and Basingstoke: Macmillan Press for International Economic Association.

WEEKS, L. E. and BERMAN, H. J. (eds) (1977) *Economics in Health Care*. Germantown, Md: Aspen.

WILLIAMS, A. (1977) 'What can Economists do to Help Health Service Planning?' pp. 301–35 in ARTIS, N. J. and NOBAY, A. R. (eds) *Studies in Modern Economic Analysis* (Proceedings of the Association of University Teachers of Economics, Edinburgh, 1976). Oxford: Basil Blackwell.

Chapter 1. Health, Doctors and Health Care Resources

On the nature of health, ill health and the contribution of health care to health, Cochrane (1972) is a thought-provoking beginning. For a highly critical stance on doctors and health care see Illich (1976). On the economics of clinical practice, e.g. diagnosis and decision-making, drugs etc., a recent collection of papers is Phillips and Wolfe (1977).

COCHRANE, A. L. (1972) *Effectiveness and Efficiency, Random Reflections on Health Services* (Rock Carling Fellowship Lecture). London: Nuffield Provincial Hospitals Trust.

ILLICH, I. (1976) *Limits to Medicine, Medical Nemisis: The Expropriation of Health*. London: Marion Boyars; also published (1977) Harmondsworth: Penguin.

PHILLIPS, C. I. and WOLFE, J. N. (eds) (1977) *Clinical Practice and Economics*. Tunbridge Wells: Pitman Medical Publishing Co.

Chapter 2. Health Care as an Economic Good

For an early succinct discussion of the characteristics that health care possesses and a discussion of their policy relevance see Lees (1962). A thorough and clear survey/analysis of the various characteristics of health care and their importance can be found in Culyer (1971). A technically easier-going discussion can be found in Culyer (1972). Wiseman (1963) also contains much interesting economic argument on the nature of health care. An economist's view of the work of Titmuss can be found in Reisman (1977).

CULYER, A. J. (1971) 'The Nature of the Commodity "Health Care" and its Efficient Allocation', *Oxford Economic Papers*, Vol. 23, No. 2 (July), pp. 189–211; reprinted as Reading 2, pp. 49–74 in COOPER, M. H. and CULYER, A. J. (eds) (1973) *Health Economics*. Harmondsworth: Penguin.

CULYER, A. J. (1972) 'The "Market" versus the "State" in Medical Care – A Minority Report on an Empty Academic Box', pp. 1–31 in McLachlan, G. (ed.) *Problems and Progress in Medical Care*; *Essays in Current Research* (7th Series). London: Oxford University Press for Nuffield Provincial Hospitals Trust.

LEES, D. (1962) 'The Logic of the British National Health Service', *Journal of Law and Economics*, Vol. 5 (October), pp. 111–18.

REISMAN, D. A. (1977) *Richard Titmuss: Welfare and Society*. London: Heinemann.

WISEMAN, J. (1963) 'Cost Benefit Analysis and Health Service Policy', *Scottish Journal of Political Economy*, Vol. 10, No. 1 (February), pp. 128–45; also pp. 433–51 in Kiker, B. F. (ed.) *Investment in Human Capital*. Columbia, South Carolina: University of South Carolina Press.

Chapter 3. Health Care and Market Intervention

The main reading on the material in this chapter are the articles (and book) cited as references to Chapter 3. However Arrow (1963) deserves and repays careful attention.

ARROW, K. J. (1963) 'Uncertainty and the Welfare Economics of Medical Care', *American Economic Review*, Vol. 53, No. 5 (December), pp. 941–73; reprinted as Reading 1, pp. 13–48 in COOPER M. H. and CULYER, A. J. (eds) (1973) *Health Economics*. Harmondsworth: Penguin.

Chapter 4. The Demand for Health Care

Grossman (1972) is the most sophisticated and complete treatment to date. Dowie (1975) provides a very good assessment, critique and extension of Grossman's work. On 'need' Williams (1974) is a very good survey and discussion.

DOWIE, J. (1975) 'The Portfolio Approach to Health Behaviour', *Social Science and Medicine*, Vol. 9, No. 11/12 (November/December), pp. 619–31.

GROSSMAN, M. (1972) *The Demand for Health: a Theoretical and Empirical Investigation* (National Bureau of Economic Research Occasional Paper 119). New York and London: Columbia University Press.

WILLIAMS, A. (1974) '"Need" as a Demand Concept (With Special Reference to Health)', Chapter 4, pp. 60–78 in CULYER, A. J. (ed.) *Economic Policies and Social Goals: Aspects of Public Choice.* London: Martin Robertson.

Chapter 5. Empirical Evidence on the Demand for Health Care

The references at the end of this chapter represent the main research on this issue; however, Ginsburg and Mannheim (1973) is a useful addition.

GINSBURG, P. B. and MANNHEIM, L. M. (1973) 'Insurance Co-payment and Health Services Utilisation: A Critical review', *Economic Business Bulletin*, Vol. 25, No. 2 pp. 142–53.

Chapter 6. The Theory of Supply

Jacobs (1974) is a very useful survey of economic models of hospitals. He divides models into 'organism' and 'exchange' categories. The former models treat hospitals as entities with their own goals, e.g. quality, quantity-maximising models. The latter models seek to identify and analyse the actions of those individuals who use the hospital as an organisation that functions to enable them to further their own ends. Feldstein (1974) also contains a survey of hospital models. A recent addition to the literature is Harris (1977).

FELDSTEIN, M. S. (1974) 'Econometric Studies of Health Economics', pp. 377–447 in INTRILLIGATOR, M. and KENDRICK, D. A. (eds) *Frontiers of Quantitative Economics II.* Amsterdam: North-Holland.

HARRIS, J. (1977) 'The Internal Organisation of Hospitals: Some Economic Implications', *The Bell Journal of Economics*, Vol. 8, No. 2 (Autumn), pp. 467–82.

JACOBS, P. (1974) 'A Survey of Economic Models of Hospitals', *Inquiry*, Vol. 11, No. 2 (June), pp. 83–97.

Chapter 7. Estimating Hospital Costs

Berki (1972), Chapter 5, is a very clear discussion of this topic. On the use of econometrics in general in health care see Feldstein (1967, 1974).

BERKI, S. E. (1972) *Hospital Economics.* Lexington, Massachusetts: Lexington Books, D. C. Heath & Co.

FELDSTEIN, M. S. (1967) *Economic Analysis for Health Service Efficiency.* Amsterdam: North-Holland.

FELDSTEIN, M. S. (1974) 'Econometric Studies of Health Economics', pp. 377–447 in INTRILLIGATOR, M. and KENDRICK, D. A. (eds) *Frontiers of Quantitative Economics II.* Amsterdam: North-Holland.

Chapter 8. Health Care, Cost – Benefit and Cost-Effectiveness Techniques

For an introduction to cost – benefit analysis (CBA) in general and a collection of some of the classic articles on the topic see Layard (1972). For a survey of applications to health care see Klarman (1974) and Roberts (1974). Williams (1974) and Williams and Anderson (1975) provide a very clear discussion of the foundations of applying CBA to health care.

KLARMAN, H. E. (1974) 'Application of Cost Benefit Analysis to Health Services and the Special Case of Technologic Innovation', *International Journal of Health Services*, Vol. 4, No. 2 (Spring), pp. 325–52.

LAYARD, R. (ed.) (1972) *Cost Benefit Analysis.* Harmondsworth: Penguin.

ROBERTS, J. A. (1974) 'Economic Evaluation of Health Care', *British Journal of Preventive and Social Medicine*, Vol. 28, No. 3 (August), pp. 210–16.

WILLIAMS, A. (1974) 'The Cost Benefit Approach', *British Medical Bulletin*, Vol. 30, No. 3 (September), pp. 252–6.

WILLIAMS, A. and ANDERSON, R. (1975) *Efficiency in the Social Services.* Oxford: Basil Blackwell; London: Martin Robertson.

Chapter 9. Valuing Human Life

On this topic Mishan (1971) is probably the best starting point. Book-length treatments of this subject are Jones Lee (1976) and Mooney (1977). Fromm (1977) provides a useful discussion of reservations relating to the 'willingness to pay approach'. Needleman (1976) is an empirical investigation of the value 'others' place on those exposed to risk of death.

FROMM, G. (1977) 'Individual and Social Preferences: Safety Regulations and Life and Injury Valuation', *Rivista Internazionale di Economic adi Transport*, Vol. 3, No. 1, pp. 3–20.

JONES LEE, M. W. (1976) *The Value of Life: An Economic Analysis.* London: Martin Robertson.

MISHAN, E. (1971) 'Evaluation of Life and Limb: A Theoretical Approach', *Journal of Political Economy*, Vol. 79, No. 4 (July/August), pp. 687–705; reprinted as Reading 8, pp. 219–42 in LAYARD, R. (ed.) (1972) *Cost Benefit Analysis.* Harmondsworth: Penguin.

MOONEY, G. H. (1977) *The Valuation of Human Life*. London and Basingstoke: Macmillan.

NEEDLEMAN, L. (1976) 'Valuing Other People's Lives', *Manchester School*, Vol. 44, No. 4 (December), pp. 309–42.

Chapter 10. Economic Aspects of a Public Health Care System: the U.K.

Cooper (1975) provides an economic overview of the nature and problems of Britain's National Health Service. A discussion of the financing and organisation of health services in the developed world can be found in Appendices D to Q in British Medical Association (1970). For a recent discussion of the case for the 'pricing' of health care services see Chapter 5 of Seldon (1977). For material on the health care systems of other European countries and the Soviet Union and East European countries see Maynard (1975) and Kaser (1976) respectively.

BRITISH MEDICAL ASSOCIATION (1970) *Health Services Financing*. London: British Medical Association.

COOPER, M. H. (1975) *Rationing Health Care*. London: Croom Helm.

KASER, M. (1976) *Health Care in the Soviet Union and Eastern Europe*. London: Croom Helm.

MAYNARD, A. (1975) *Health Care in the European Community*. London: Croom Helm.

SELDON, A. (1977) *Charge*. London: Maurice Temple Smith.

Chapter 11. Economic Aspects of a Private Health Care System: the U.S.

Sorkin (1975) is a text essentially devoted to the US health care system, as is Ward (1975). Papers and comments that use a lot of the arguments discussed in Chapters 1, 2, 3 and 11 in an interesting discussion of demands for national health insurance in the United States are Fuchs (1976), Moore (1976) and Munch (1976).

FUCHS, V. R. (1976) 'From Bismarck to Woodcock: The 'Irrational' Pursuit of National Health Insurance', *Journal of Law and Economics*, Vol. 19, No. 2 (August), pp. 347–59.

MOORE, T. G. (1976) 'From Bismarck to Woodcock: The 'Irrational' Pursuit of National Health Insurance: Comment', *Journal of Law and Economics*, Vol. 19, No. 2 (August), pp. 360–3.

MUNCH, P. (1976) 'From Bismarck to Woodcock: The 'Irrational' Pursuit of National Health Insurance: Comment', *Journal of Law and Economics*, Vol. 19, No. 2 (August), pp. 365–9.

SORKIN, A. L. (1975) *Health Economics.* Lexington, Massachusetts: Lexington Books, D. C. Heath & Co.
WARD, R. A. (1975) *The Economics of Health Resources.* Reading, Massachusetts: Addison-Wesley.

Chapter 12. Economic Aspects of a Developing Health Care System

A recent book especially devoted to this subject is Sorkin (1976). Chapters 9 and 11 of Abel-Smith (1976) contain much interesting material on health care and health care planning in developing countries.

ABEL-SMITH, B. (1976) *Value for Money in Health Services.* London: Heinemann.
SORKIN, A. L. (1976) *Health Care in Developing Countries.* Lexington, Massachusetts: Lexington Books, D. C. Heath & Co.

Author Index

Subject Index